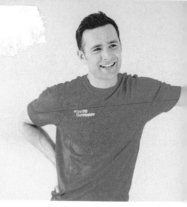

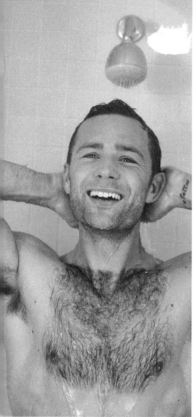

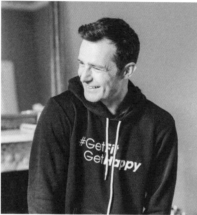

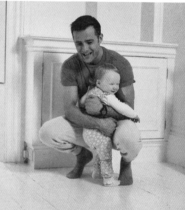

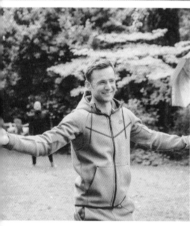

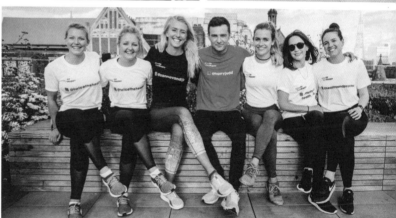

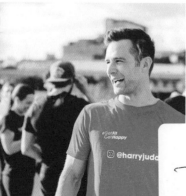

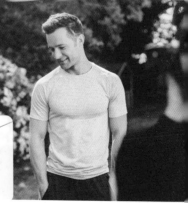

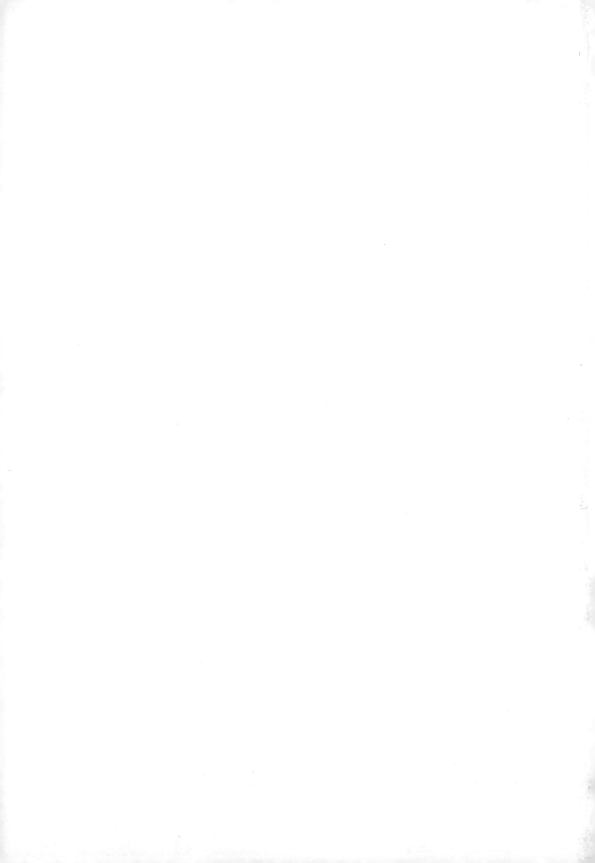

GET FIT, GET HAPPY

First published in Great Britain in 2017 by Coronet, an imprint of Hodder & Stoughton
An Hachette UK company

2

A CIP catalogue record for this title is available from the British Library

Trade Paperback ISBN: 978 1 473 64873 9
Ebook ISBN: 978 1 473 64874 6

**The information herein is not intended to replace the services of trained health
and fitness professionals, or be a substitute for medical advice. If you have any
concerns regarding your fitness or health you should first consult with a medical
professional before starting in any exercise programme. Always consider your
own ability before doing any of the workouts in this book.**

Publisher: Charlotte Hardman
Photographer: Dan Jones
Design: Nathan Burton
Shoot Producer: Ruth Ferrier
Stylist: Rosalind Keep
Fitness Consultant: Adam Jones
Copyeditor: Julia Kellaway

Colour origination by Born Group

Printed and bound in Germany by Mohn Media

Hodder & Stoughton policy is to use papers that are natural, renewable and recyclable
products and made from wood grown in sustainable forests. The logging and manufacturing
processes are expected to conform to the environmental regulations of the country of origin.

Hodder & Stoughton Ltd
Carmelite House
50 Victoria Embankment
London EC4Y 0DZ

www.hodder.co.uk

GET FIT,
GET HAPPY

HARRY JUDD

CORONET

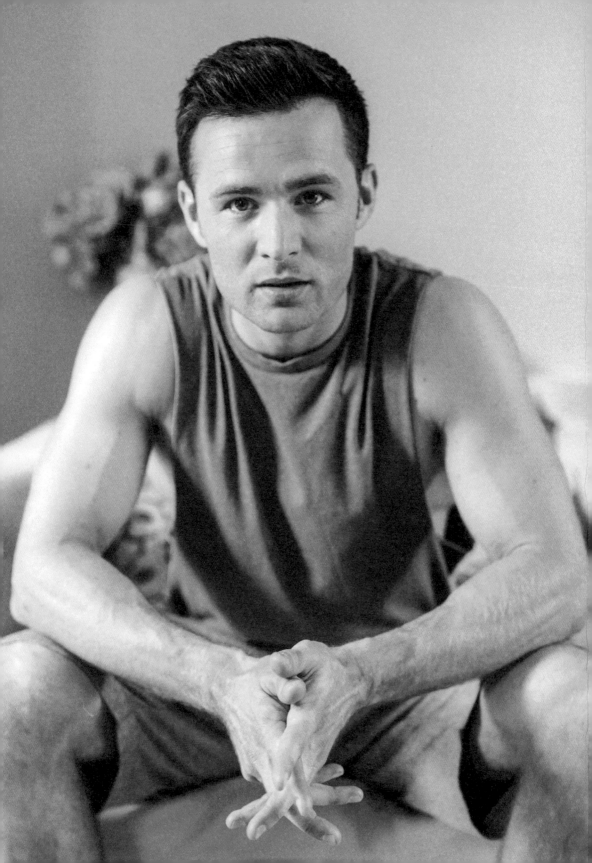

CONTENTS

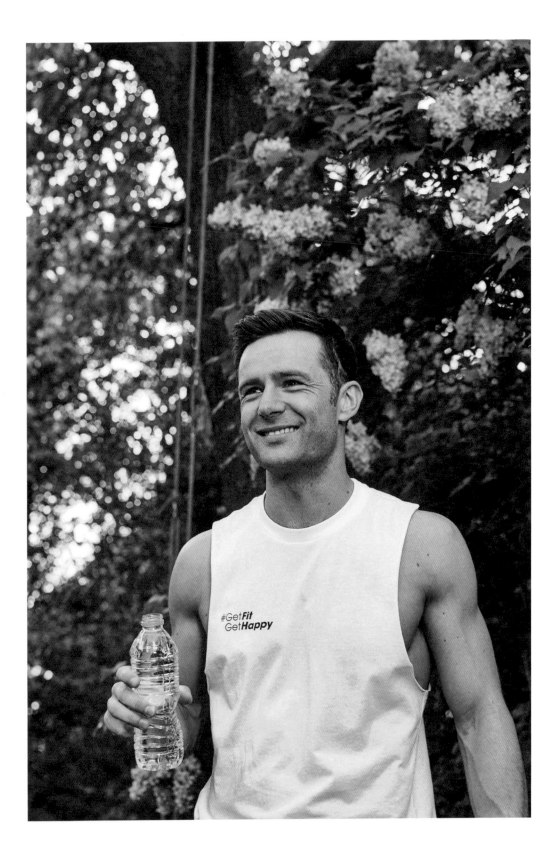

INTRODUCTION

This is the story of how exercise turned my life around. It's done that not because it's made me fitter, or because it's made me healthier, or because it's made me leaner and stronger – although all these things are true. It's turned my life around because it's made me feel better. I think it can make you feel better too.

We all know we should exercise, but so many of us don't. And although I am a self-confessed fitness fanatic, I totally get why people don't exercise. Many people find exercise intimidating and they worry that they don't have the time or money to make a commitment to it.

I'd like to show you that in order to exercise effectively, you can do it anywhere: in the kitchen, the park, the gym, the office etc. You can do it with friends, family, colleagues or by yourself but you certainly don't need anything else. It can be simple and it should always be fun.

I want to change the way people think about exercise. I want to encourage people to start exercising not because it will get them ripped or turning heads, but because of the one positive benefit that anyone can reap, no matter how fit they are, no matter how old they are, no matter what shape or size they are.

I WANT TO GET PEOPLE EXERCISING BECAUSE IT MAKES THEM FEEL EPIC.

In fact, I'd go even further than that. As anyone who has ever encountered difficulties with their mood (and that's a lot of us, right?) probably knows, all doctors and health professionals encourage exercise as a means of treating everything from anxiety to panic attacks to depression. In many instances, exercise can be as effective an intervention as medication and talking therapies.

But my philosophy is for anyone who, for whatever reason, finds that they sometimes need a bit of a boost in their mood. It is not just for those who have diagnosed mental health difficulties. Everyone has ups and downs in their lives. I firmly believe that a little regular exercise can go a very long way to helping us deal with those moments when life feels like it's getting on top of us; those moments when we're feeling blue, stressed, tired or just a bit out of sorts.

The bottom line is this: exercise can be awesome!

I want to encourage you not to worry about expensive gym memberships and fancy exercise gear. I want to persuade you that getting into exercise does not mean you have to devote to it massive chunks of time that you simply don't have. For some people, the aesthetic benefits of exercise are a motivating factor, and that's fine. But if that's not you, I want to steer you away from social media sites where guys and girls post pictures of their perfect glutes that you find positively demotivating. I'm not saying you won't look great if you start exercising, but

OUR MEASUREMENT ISN'T GOING TO BE THE SIZE OF OUR BICEPS. IT'S GOING TO BE THE SIZE OF OUR SMILES.

Because whoever we are, from whatever walk of life, I believe that exercise has the power to make everything seem better.

I'm aware that perhaps that sounds strange coming from someone who has the best job in the world, who lives his life in the public eye and who perhaps seems to 'have it all'. Fair point. I'm not going to pretend life hasn't been good to me. I left school at the age of 17 to join McFly, which would become one of the biggest pop acts in the country. I have spent my adult life playing to packed arenas of fans screaming so loudly I have sometimes found it hard to hear my own drums above the noise. I have toured the UK and the world. I became a regular TV fixture in the living rooms of millions of people when I competed on, and won, *Strictly Come Dancing*. I met the love of my life. We have a beautiful family. From the outside looking in, my life has been great. More than that: it's been charmed. You'll never hear me utter a word of complaint about the hand I've been dealt.

But lives are complicated things. They are full of light and shade, of mountains and valleys. In that sense, mine is no different to a life that hasn't been lived in the public eye. In fact, I'll be willing to bet, mine has probably not been that much different to yours.

This book begins with that thought. Over the years, like everyone, I've had my share of difficulties to overcome. From the outset, I want to be completely honest about those difficulties, how they've affected me and the strategies I've developed to cope with them. By the time you've finished reading these pages, you'll hopefully understand the massive effect exercise has had on my life and on my ability to deal with certain

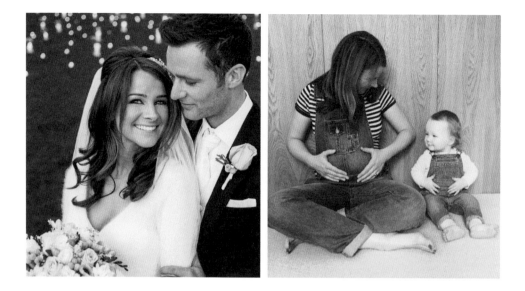

problems. Some of these problems have been self-inflicted and of my own making, and I accept full responsibility for that. Others, I suspect, have been dormant inside me for a long time, as they are with many people.

Whatever the truth, I find these issues extremely difficult to talk about. We live in a world where it's increasingly acceptable to talk openly about mental health. It's great to see that people are, little by little, becoming more confident in admitting to themselves and to others that they're struggling. But it hasn't always been that way. In the throes of my own anxiety, I've had my share of people telling me to 'man up', not understanding quite what I was going through. And if you're anything like me, you'll know how tough it can be to speak up about these matters.

I've only ever shared some of what you're about to read with those closest to me. I am writing about my memories and feelings here not because I want sympathy. I don't. I know that plenty of people have it worse than me. By the same token, I know that there are many people who struggle to admit that they occasionally suffer from feeling anxious, down, stressed or on edge. I hope that, in sharing my experiences, in explaining for the first time where they come from and what I do to deal with them, I might help people who need a bit of a boost.

SO. DEEP BREATH. HERE GOES ...

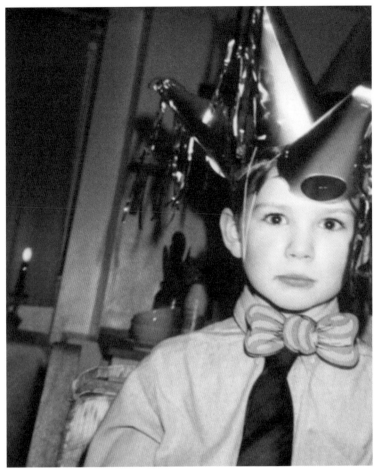
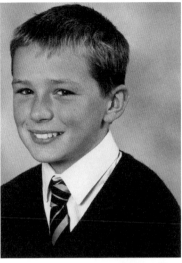
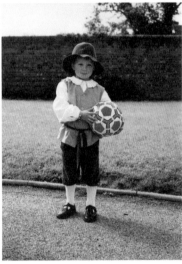
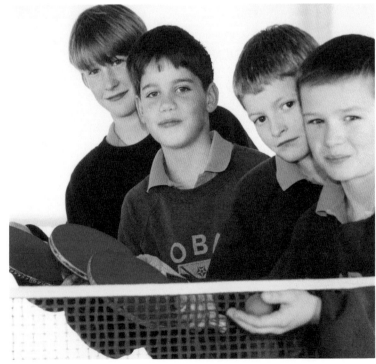
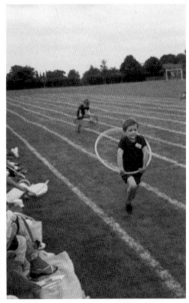

MESSING WITH MY HEAD

I'm a happy, upbeat adult, and I was a happy, upbeat kid. So upbeat, in fact, that I was a bit of a handful – always full of energy, always wanting to be outside in the fresh air and never happier than when I had a ball to kick around or a cricket bat in my hands. My mum always says I was forever vaulting out of my cot, and that I'd clambered to the top of the climbing frame by the time I was one. If truth be told, I was a bit hyper and overemotional. I couldn't stay still and it was by all accounts a nightmare trying to get me to do my homework! I guess I was your regular, tearaway little boy (and some would say that not much has changed …)

When I was seven, my parents were involved in a bad car accident. For my mum, it was a case of history horribly repeating itself, because her brother had been killed in a similarly terrible car crash. Dad suffered minor injuries, but Mum broke both her ankles and her left arm, and dislocated both her shoulders. She was in a wheelchair for a year. Happily, she came through it. But having to cope with a hyperactive seven-year-old at the time was just too much for her. It had always been the intention that I'd go to a good local school, but Mum's condition after the car accident pushed my parents to make a different decision for me. I was sent to boarding school at the age of eight, along with my brother, who was ten at the time. My sister, who is four years older than me, went to a girls' boarding school.

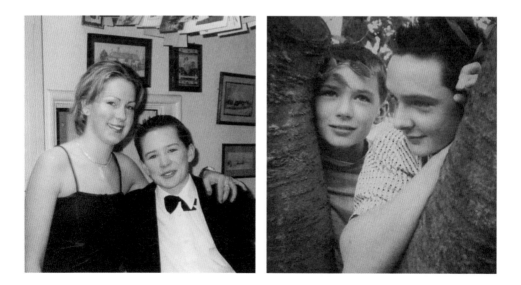

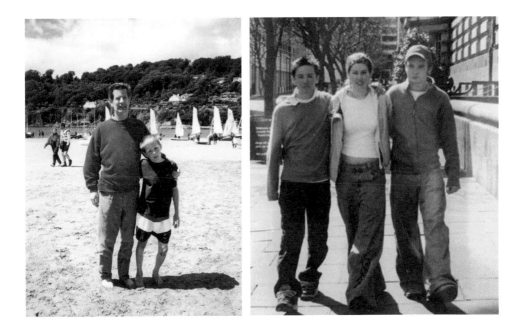

One of the first times I remember feeling truly nervous was when my mum and dad took me to school that first day. We were always a very close, loving family, and it was daunting to know that I was about to be separated from my mum and dad.

Those memories are burned into my brain. The guys in the band always joke that my school sounds a bit like Hogwarts. They're not far wrong. I remember trundling up that huge driveway in the middle of nowhere and walking through the huge oak doors into the enormous oak hallway, clutching my tuck box with the headmaster looking over me. I recall seeing my dad with a tear in his eye, then looking round and realising that my parents had gone because the teachers preferred it that way: no long, drawn-out goodbyes.

In reality, however, my time at boarding school was not some Charles Dickens-like nightmare. I loved it.

BOARDING SCHOOL WAS THE PERFECT PLACE FOR ME. I GOT TO CHARGE AROUND ALL DAY LONG, BEFORE CRASHING, EXHAUSTED, INTO BED.

I was surrounded by my mates, I had access to a drum kit and, perhaps even more importantly to me at that time, to the playing fields. My time at boarding school was character-building and made me much more independent than I perhaps would have been otherwise. I understand that it wouldn't be right for plenty of people. Certainly, now that I'm a father, I'd find it pretty tough to be separated from my children for weeks on end. But for me, back then, boarding school was completely the right call. I enjoyed every minute of it.

My point is this: the anxiety I would later suffer was not a result of an unhappy childhood or of some deep-seated, lingering resentment at being sent away from home. I was your regular, boisterous, happy kid, from a loving family, given every advantage. I was very lucky.

I was also, I think, keen to be seen as the cool kid. I was a bit of a rebel: naughty, but with a knack of knowing how to get away with it. That was probably why, at the age of 16 or 17, just as I was getting into bands, drinking and smoking when I should have been studying, I began to dabble with marijuana.

It wasn't very serious, at least it didn't seem so at the time. How could it be? All my friends were quite adamant that the weed we were smoking was non-addictive. Really it was just a bit of fun. We'd do it mostly in the school holidays, round at each other's houses, hanging out with a joint after our parents had gone to bed. It was weak stuff and we didn't really see any harm in it.

And then came McFly.

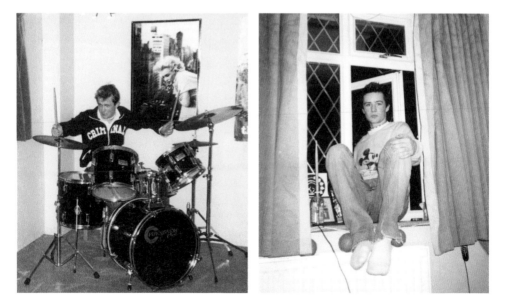

A mate of mine, in an attempt to get his music career going, had headed to London to play for a guy who managed one of the biggest bands at the time: Busted. My friend found out that the manager was looking for a drummer and bass player for a new band he was putting together. I decided to go for the audition. I needed my parents' permission first, and Mum was a bit reluctant. There were more important things to consider, like school and university. But my dad put her mind at rest: 'Harry will *never* get into that band,' he told her!

There was a queue of people outside the audition room and, although I did my best to look confident, I was as nervous as hell inside. When I was asked if I could sing and play the drums at the same time, I brazenly said that was no problem. In fact,

MY VOCAL PERFORMANCE OF BUSTED'S 'YEAR 3000' IN THAT AUDITION WAS ABOUT THE MOST CRINGEY THING I'D EVER DONE.

However, while I wasn't the best drummer at that audition, I wasn't the worst. Through a mixture of drumming and feigned confidence, I got down to the last two.

The final round of auditions took place over a couple of days. My rival was a better drummer than me, but perhaps a bit more straight-laced. I decided to do what I was best at and concentrate on getting on with everybody. My outward show of confidence got me through. I was in.

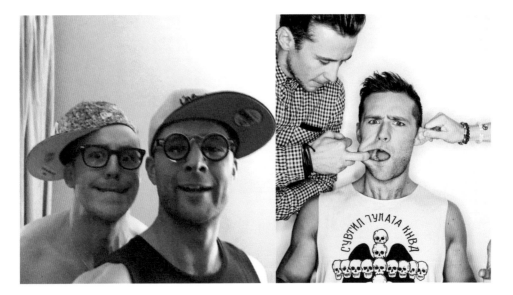

Joining McFly meant leaving school. A big call, and although to me it was a no-brainer, my parents weren't keen. They wanted me to get my A levels and go to university, and I can certainly understand their anxiety. But I was desperate to be a part of this exciting new opportunity and in the end my mum and dad gave it their blessing.

So I dropped out of school, joined McFly and found myself living in a fantastic band house with three new best friends: Tom, Danny and Dougie.

I had money in my pocket and fame was just around the corner. Life was sweet, and I felt like I was doing it justice.

Too much justice, perhaps.

Even as early as the auditions for the band, I had wondered whether tales of the rock 'n' roll lifestyle were true, and whether smoking would become a more permanent fixture in my life. It did. Away from the watchful eyes of school and parents, I became a much more regular smoker.

In the early days of McFly, we had quite the clean-cut image. We didn't like to think of ourselves as a regular 'boy band', as we wrote our own songs and played our own instruments. But, as with the more manufactured boy bands, a certain level of behaviour was expected of us by our management. Behind the scenes, however, things were a bit different, my room in the band house was thick with the fog of marijuana smoke.

I'm hoping that by the time you reach the end of this story you'll come to the same conclusion as me – that getting involved with illegal substances of any kind is a bad idea whether you're of an anxious frame of mind or not. But I'm going to tell you the truth: I loved my weed. Smoking was a daily occurrence. Sure, being out there with the band was a blast, but even when I was playing to thousands and lapping up the adulation of the fans, it always felt good returning to the band house so I could roll up and spark up. To me, it became a part of life.

When our manager Fletch caught us smoking and quite rightly read us the riot act, we promised to kick it. Some of the others did, but I didn't. This was the worst mistake of my life.

People make light of marijuana use, and maybe it's true that the weed and resin I'd started out on was less damaging, but I wasn't using that any more. It just didn't give me the kick I was after. I was on the hard stuff – a few puffs of it and you'd be away with the fairies. Sounds fun? Not really. I remembered how my friends had told me that marijuana was not addictive. I hadn't been on the skunk for very long before I realised that this simply wasn't true.

Despite all the other amazing things that were happening to me – and they *were* amazing – weed was really all I could think about. I had been given the opportunity of a lifetime, but my constant priority was to go home and get stoned. Deep down, I knew it was becoming a problem. There were moments when I would think to myself, 'I am never going to be able to stop doing this.' It seemed impossible. I couldn't sleep without it; I couldn't really function without it. I was quite sure back then that I'd be smoking weed forever. I used to think that all I wanted in life was a flat in London with my own private balcony, so I could sit there and smoke all day long. Sad, I know, given all the other opportunities that were in front of me, but true.

I had a girlfriend at the time. She had been in the year above me at school. Her dad was in the army, stationed in Canada. We'd been an item for about a year and a half when I flew to Canada to see her. This was the first time since being on the skunk that I'd had an enforced absence from it. It was horrible. I remember a terrible feeling in my stomach, a gnawing kind of ache. I thought there was something physically wrong with me, but I just didn't know what it could be. I didn't particularly associate this feeling with my sudden abstinence. I even told my girlfriend and her mum that I had something wrong with my tummy.

I REALISE NOW, HOWEVER, THAT I WAS SUFFERING FROM THE PHYSICAL EFFECTS OF ANXIETY AND PARANOIA.

I had never experienced that feeling before. I couldn't identify it and I certainly didn't know how to deal with it.

My solution, I suppose, was entirely predictable. Having said goodbye to my girlfriend at the end of my stay, I flew back into London, went straight back to the band house, picked up some skunk, rolled a joint and sparked up. Immediately, the feeling in my stomach went away. My poison was also my medicine.

I hated travelling in those early days of McFly, not because I was homesick, but because it meant I couldn't have any weed. No weed meant anxiety, and no sleep. It caused tensions. Arguments. We would be travelling to some amazing place and I'd be putting a dampener on the proceedings simply because I couldn't get stoned. Unable to sleep, I'd be tired the next morning, then further exhausted by full days of interviews. It made me very grumpy.

I should have stopped there and then, of course. But that didn't seem to be an option. I told myself that I enjoyed it too much. The truth was that I was simply hooked. So instead of taking a step back, I took several steps forward – because that would make me enjoy it more, right? I decided I'd have a couple of beers before smoking a joint, but a couple soon became four or five as I looked for ways to increase the high. Smoking was starting to take over my life; the more I smoked, the more anxious I became. The knot in my stomach became a regular morning thing. More than that, I began to experience crippling panic attacks, which started to affect my ability to do my job.

Let me make myself clear: these experiences are no different to the experiences of lots of people who find that dabbling with drugs is a bad idea. However, when you are in the public eye, these problems can be amplified.

In 2005, McFly were due to attend the Brit Awards, where we were nominated for Best Pop Act. My anxiety and panic attacks had been getting worse and worse in the days leading up to the awards ceremony. The weed I was smoking was making them worse, but I was so hooked on the stuff that I simply couldn't stop, even though I knew I should.

The night arrived. It's anxiety-inducing being on the red carpet at the best of times. The state I was in, the last thing I wanted was to have all eyes on me, cameras flashing, people shouting. I felt like passing out. And although I desperately wanted to enjoy myself that night, to revel in what we'd achieved as a band, all I could think was that I would give up everything we had with a click of my fingers, if it would only make my anxiety disappear. When Jodie Kidd announced that we had won the award for Best Pop Act, I was terrified at the prospect of having to go up there to accept it. As a band we are, at the best of times, a bit uncomfortable in 'red carpet' situations – it's probably something to do with being the focus of so many people's attention. But the pressure of this particular event, the enormity of the thing, got to me. Walking up to get that award, I felt crushed with anxiety.

Somehow I jumped that hurdle, but then I had the aftershow to negotiate. People kept coming up to congratulate me, to ask me how I was. I told them I was fine. I wasn't. In fact, I wanted to break down in front of them. I remember meeting Robbie Williams and thinking, 'Hey, he's had some drug problems. Maybe he can give me some advice.' But it wasn't the time or place for a paranoid conversation like that. I had to keep my problems to myself. I couldn't tell anyone.

I was, quite frankly, an anxious, panic-stricken mess.

I needed quiet and space to sort my head out, but that simply wasn't possible. There was no let-up in our schedule. Three days after the Brit Awards we flew, along with our manager Fletch, to New Orleans, where we were due to spend three weeks filming for a major Hollywood movie called *Just My Luck*. In the movie, McFly were to play a band in search of the big time, but who were stuck with a super-unlucky manager played by Chris Pine. It should have been a blast, but by the time we arrived in New Orleans, my anxiety was no better. I felt like I'd never be well again.

I was desperate. I couldn't bottle it in any longer. I knew I had to talk to someone about what I was going through. When we arrived in America, I sat down with my band mates and explained to them how I was feeling. 'Guys, something's seriously wrong with me. I'm not sure I can stay out here. I'm not sure I can do the movie.'

I was met with stunned silence. Looking back, I can understand their surprise. They were so used to seeing the confident, outgoing Harry, the Harry who always took everything in his stride, that the existence of this anxious, crippled, terrified Harry must have been a shock to them. Then I dropped another bombshell: 'I'm going to have to tell Fletch.'

They tried to talk me out of it, which I completely understood. Over the years, we would all support each other through our ups and downs, and do what we could to be there for each other. But I knew why they were nervous. Fletch had drawn a line in the sand a year before when it came to marijuana use. We'd promised him that we would stay on the right side of it. I'd betrayed his trust and the band was going to suffer. The guys were scared of what he'd say and do. *I* was scared of what he'd say and do. But I was even more scared of the terrible anxiety I was experiencing.

I found Fletch. We sat in his hotel room, my heart thumping in my chest as I tried to take control of my nerves. I was on the edge of tears, and obviously so.

'Harry, what is it?'

I told him everything about my anxiety, my panic attacks and what had caused them. When I had finished, I sat with my head hung, staring at the floor, waiting for him to give me both barrels and tell me I was out of the band.

But he didn't.

Fletch was brilliant. He became my confidant over the following days and weeks. For the first time since being in McFly I felt I couldn't talk to the other guys. They were having the best time, hanging out in New Orleans, filming a movie. I understood. I couldn't rain on their parade. We were in the prime of our lives, supposedly having the time of our lives. But while they were flying high, I was an anxious mess. I didn't want to drag them down with me, but nor did I expect them to understand just how terrible I was feeling. I spent the whole time talking to Fletch. Talking and talking. Opening up. I barely left his side. He soon came to the realisation that I was quite seriously ill. He told me that I could get on a plane back to the UK immediately, that my health was more important than anything and that they'd find me a replacement in the movie so I could concentrate on getting better.

As bad as I felt, and as desperate as I was, I made the decision not to do that. Deep down, I was angry with myself for this self-inflicted situation I was in. I told myself I had to suck it up and get through the next few weeks, somehow. Looking back, I think it was the right call. But it meant I had a super-tough few weeks ahead of me.

In *Just My Luck* there's a scene where Harry the drummer gets lost just before the gig – it's the climax of the film. Harry is backstage twiddling with his sticks, when he drops one. It falls beneath the stage, so he goes down to retrieve it. The trapdoor shuts and Harry's shut in. He's calling out to everyone, trying to be let out. He finds some buttons to press, the floor rises up and he's suddenly on stage, surrounded by dry ice. I'm not going to lie, it's pretty cringey stuff when I look back on it. It also brings back a horrible memory of the day we filmed it.

Something about the dry ice and the confined space made me freak out. A mad feeling of uncontrollable panic rose in my gut. My heart was pumping like a drum. I was sweating. I felt trapped in my own skin. I was overcome with an all-consuming urge to get out of there, to be somewhere else. I sprinted off set, without explaining anything to anyone.

The studio was on a busy road, on the other side of which was a car park where the McFly trailer was situated. I sprinted across that road, barely aware of the traffic, horns beeping at me from left and right. I burst into our trailer. My band mate Danny was there, and thank goodness. I sat in his arms while he did what he could to calm me down as the panic attack passed. When I subsequently watched that scene at the film's premiere, it's not my dodgy mullet that grabs my attention, it's the memory of how I was feeling. Nobody else would know – but I could see it all in my eyes.

Somehow I made it through the filming process. It was a very surreal experience, not only because of my fragile mental state, but also because of a certain young starlet by the name of Lindsay Lohan taking a shine to me (a long story, which I won't go into here!). I was in a constant state of worry that the press would somehow find out about my panic attacks. It was the most anxiety-inducing thought ever. Of course, it was easier to keep things secret in those days, when not everybody had a smartphone in their pocket. But when a paparazzi photographer took a shot of me in tears sitting with Fletch, and the paper wrote that I was homesick, we didn't comment on the real reason for my distress. But I wasn't homesick. I wasn't just sick.

But I wasn't homesick. I was just sick. I saw an American doctor and explained everything. He prescribed me some Valium, but I didn't want to take it. I didn't really know what Valium was, but I was loath to put anything into my body that remotely resembled a drug, because it might make things worse. A week later we had a few days off. We went to Disney World. While the guys were off enjoying themselves, I stayed with Fletch in my hotel room, freaking out. He persuaded me to try taking one of the pills. As soon as I swallowed the pill, panic hit – the familiar burning in my stomach, the raised heartbeat. 'Fletch,' I breathed, 'it's happening … please … stay with me …'

With the benefit of hindsight, I should have known that this reaction was all in my mind. But just because something's happening in your mind, it doesn't mean it's any less real. Eventually, the Valium kicked in. I felt myself calming down. Relaxing. I even felt up to walking round Disney World. Maybe everything was going to be okay.

Eventually the effects of the Valium wore off and my anxiety returned. I then read about how addictive Valium could be, and I certainly didn't want another narcotic dependence, so I didn't take it again. I looked elsewhere for ways of treating myself. I had heard someone say that orange juice was good for the chemical balance in your brain. I've never drunk so much orange juice in my life – it was my one rider demand – but, of course, it did no good.

I struggled to the end of the film shoot with my mental health showing no sign of improvement. And when we landed at Heathrow at the beginning of March 2005, I didn't even go home. I went straight to the Priory to speak to a doctor whom I prayed might be able to help me.

I sat in a consulting room with this doctor, my nerves grating, my fingernails dug into my palms, sweating profusely as I spoke solidly for ten minutes, explaining everything about my anxiety and my panic attacks. When I'd finished, the doctor nodded. 'The first thing you need to know,' he said, perfectly calm and reassuring, 'is that you're going to be absolutely fine.'

The relief was so intense that I started crying.

He asked me questions. What drugs had I been taking? How many joints had I been smoking a day? I was too scared to tell him the truth.

'One or two a day,' I said.

He looked at me.

I squirmed.

'Six a day?' I muttered.

He nodded. Then he explained that the skunk I'd been smoking had been very strong and very bad for me. It was triggering my episodes of anxiety and panic. He prescribed some antidepressant medication that would help me and assigned a therapist to my case.

'And Harry?' he added.

'Yeah?'

'No more drugs.'

I didn't need telling twice. I would do anything to feel better again. From that day to this, I haven't touched drugs even once.

The long-term effects of messing with my head, however, did not disappear along with my habit.

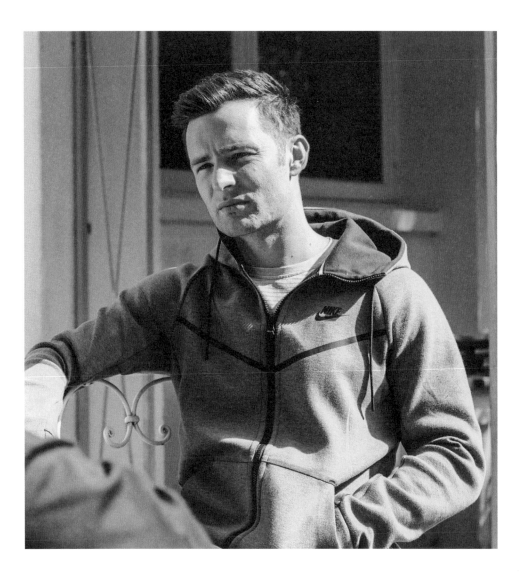

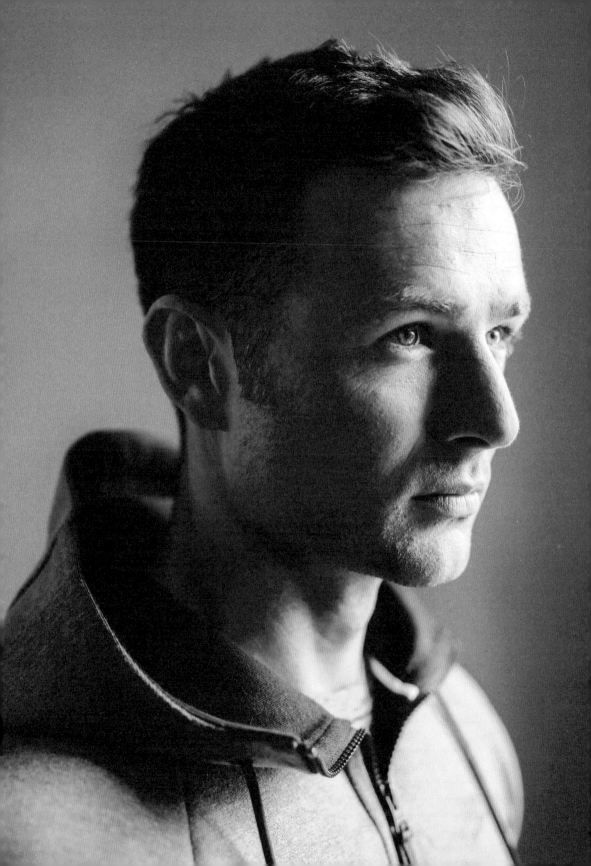

ANXIOUS HARRY

Mental health issues can be frightening. They are frightening for lots of reasons. They often have no physical manifestations – you can seldom tell by looking at someone that they are suffering from anxiety or depression, or any of the other illnesses that can affect our mental state. They aren't often talked about and they can come out of nowhere. As I've already explained, I was a confident, outgoing, happy-go-lucky teenager. When I realised that I was suffering from a mental health issue it was a shock. It didn't take long for me to appreciate, however, that these issues are far more common than I had previously understood.

When I left the Priory on my return from America, I went straight back to the band house where my brother, who is two years older than me, was waiting. I literally fell into his arms. At that time, I felt that he was one of the few people I could fully confide in. I certainly wasn't quite ready to tell my parents. My mum had known for a while that I had been dabbling with weed – it wasn't hard to miss. From time to time she'd walk into a haze of smoke when my brother and I were hanging out at home. And having resisted taking the dog for a walk for years, we had suddenly become extremely keen dog-walkers, who would come back from their new-found activity only to raid the fridge! She was, of course, not thrilled about it. She used to send me articles from the newspapers explaining the negative health effects of marijuana and had made it quite clear that, although she would always be there for us no matter what, she would find it incredibly difficult if I ever suffered any mental health issues on account of my drug use. She was a nurse. She'd seen too many people mess themselves up because of drugs.

So my first port of call was my brother. We sat in my room as I explained everything to him. After a couple of hours he said, 'You know, Harry, I've been struggling recently too.'

'Why?' I asked him.

With that simple question, he broke down in tears. 'I've just been thinking some very dark thoughts,' he said, and he described to me what I now understand to be the symptoms of anxiety and depression. It's an illness that is, I've learned, far more common in young men than we have previously been comfortable admitting. Certainly my brother has now struggled for most of his adult life. And with the benefit of hindsight, it's not surprising that this should be the case. It's a condition that is prevalent in my family. Close relatives of mine have suffered major psychotic episodes. Terence Judd, a child prodigy classical pianist, committed suicide at Beachy Head when he was 22 years of age, unable to cope with the pressure of all the expectations on him, or with his depression. My sister has suffered episodes of anxiety and my mum, who is a very emotional, open, bubbly, uplifting person, has had plenty to deal with in her life, and has had to endure the lows that come with it. You might say that it's there in my gene pool.

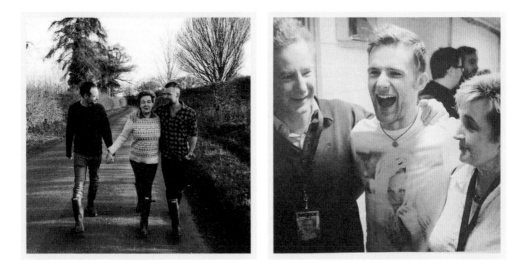

The following day I told my parents what had happened. Mum was incredibly upset. Dad was great. They drove to London and took me out for a meal. I had a panic attack while I was in the restaurant with them. As we were sitting in the car on the way back from the restaurant, the song 'Ferry Cross the Mersey' by Gerry and the Pacemakers came on the radio. It was a song from my childhood that my dad used to play – I'd loved it when I was five years old. It triggered something inside me when I heard it all those years later and I burst into tears.

Over the months that followed, Mum and Dad were incredibly supportive. I went home for a bit, whenever we had some time off. My panic attacks didn't disappear immediately. However, the antidepressant medication I was given did help and, as the doctor predicted, I slowly started to recover, even though the medication made me put on weight and affected my libido. It took a good three or four months – and many ups and downs – before I started feeling like myself again.

But I wasn't totally well. For two years I had been living life through a filter of weed-induced relaxation, followed by the help of my medication to keep me mellow. Now, however, I had nothing to calm me down. I was exposed to the reality of emotions and I finally had to accept that I wasn't good at dealing with them. I still smoked tobacco, and drank alcohol every now and then, but I didn't have any way to quash the sinister feelings of stress and anxiety that seemed to lurk in my stomach and bubble under my skin. I felt unsettled, uncomfortable with everything. That sensation of being completely chilled eluded me. My anxiety was ever-present.

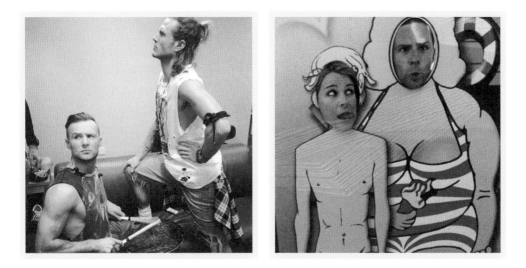

Anxiety is different to nervousness. As a performer, I was well used to the latter. Nervousness before a big show could sometimes induce laughter. There was no problem admitting to a few nerves and they could sometimes even sharpen your performance. Anxiety is a whole other proposition. More intense. Higher up the scale. More difficult to talk about and with no side benefits. It doesn't make you better at anything. Instead it cripples you.

In 2005 I met Izzy. She was playing violin in the orchestra for our *Wonderland* tour, and we first kissed in Cardiff on the penultimate night of the tour. Once the tour was over, she came to visit me in the band house and we joked that she never left. I remember telling her, with absolute certainty, that one day we would get married. Izzy was understandably wary of such a pronouncement from a 19-year-old pop drummer, but I was completely sure about what I was saying. We became an item and it was the start of the most important relationship in my life. Without Izzy, who knows where I'd be now.

The road wasn't smooth, however. I was trying to deal with this constant state of anxiety, and I think that in those early days of our relationship, I could really be quite

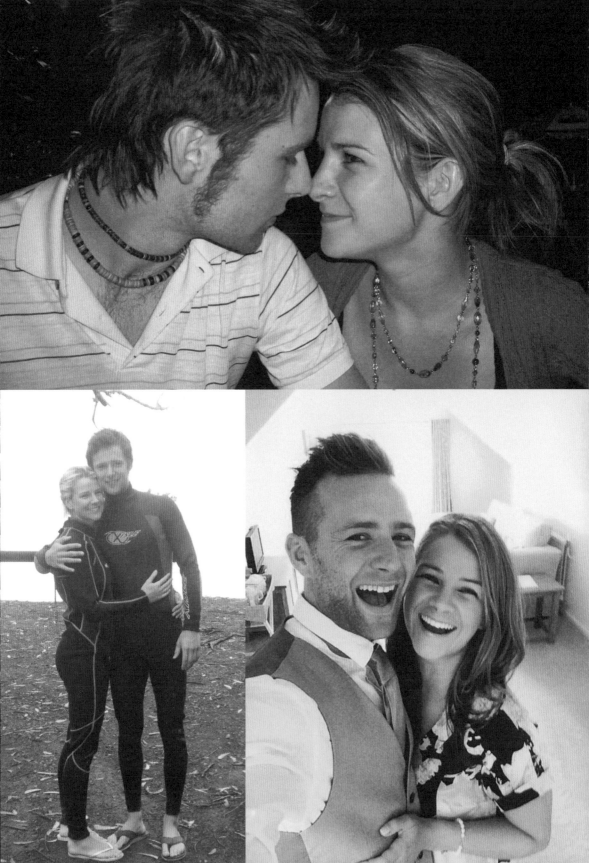

hard work. I was needy. I had quite a temper at times and my anxiety caused me to react hotly and easily fly off the handle. I wasn't dealing very well with the stresses that came with my job. We were so busy as a band and had very little time off. It wasn't that I didn't enjoy it, but sometimes I felt under enormous pressure. I know it might sound ridiculous, but I was a bit jealous of some of my mates who were at university, messing around and having fun. Sometimes the schedule and the strains of being in the public eye got on top of me.

In truth, however, I don't think I'd have been much different if I hadn't been in the public eye. I found that the underlying anxiety that caused these reactions would be triggered by ordinary situations that made it far worse.

At times when my anxiety would be triggered by emotional events, I found myself becoming completely controlled by my anxiety. It negatively informed every decision I made, or tried to make. I felt weak, constantly worried and unable to cope with anything with which life presented me. I didn't see a doctor – I think I just somehow assumed that this was what life was like – but this was extreme. I found myself crying uncontrollably. I was constantly down. My sleep was interrupted – I'd wake at exactly the same time in the small hours of the morning, every single night, and be unable to get back off again. I was short-tempered. I wouldn't talk to the guys at soundcheck. I didn't even want to be at work. On tour, I couldn't cope with being around our fans. I seriously considered quitting the band. Most of all, I needed Izzy. I remember trying to persuade her that I should leave McFly and that we should run away from it all, and buy a house in the country where the two of us could be alone and happy, away from the horrible pressures of real life.

A lot of my close friends found it hard to understand my attitude. And I don't really blame them. Confident, successful Harry had been replaced by this nervous, delicate wreck. They told me to snap out of it. To man up. To chill. They were trying to help and, of course, it was no help at all.

Eventually, my first episode of triggered anxiety subsided. I moved on and normal life resumed. The anxiety was still there in the background, however. From time to time, it flared up again. On one of these occasions I did consult a doctor, who put me back on to medication for my anxiety and asked me to try cognitive behavioural therapy (CBT). I went through the motions with CBT, but once the medication kicked in and I got back on an even keel, I didn't feel the need to continue with the therapy.

It wasn't until I was in my mid-twenties, however, that I realised there were other triggers lurking beneath the surface of my anxiety.

As I moved through my early twenties, alcohol became a bit more of a thing. It was never a real problem – I guess I was just vicariously living out my uni years throughout my twenties. The guys in the band would drink a bit, too. No more than anyone else on a big night out or enjoying university life but we'd go on tour and drink. Go abroad and drink. I'd hook up with my friends and drink. In the end, I was drinking quite heavily.

Being in a band, especially when you are young and riding high, means there are plenty of opportunities to party. We'd been playing a show in Glasgow one night. I got hammered after the gig, managed only a couple of hours' sleep, woke up the next day still drunk and continued to drink on the plane home. Back in London I met up with friends and continued this impromptu bender until five o'clock the next morning. I remember waking up at about nine o'clock, feeling absolutely terrible, having arranged to meet Izzy for a pub lunch. I clambered in to a taxi, horribly hungover, and made the date. While Izzy and I were sitting in the pub, however, I suddenly, unexpectedly found myself poleaxed by anxiety and in the midst of a crippling panic attack.

I went to see the same doctor who I'd seen after I returned from America. He explained that my anxiety could be triggered by alcohol. I needed to stop drinking.

I couldn't quite get my head round this idea. When Christmas time came around a couple of months later, feeling fine and in the Christmas spirit, I thought I'd try a couple of cheeky drinks. The anxiety kicked in. I couldn't believe it. I didn't want to believe it. Having to say to my friends that I couldn't go out for a beer? I didn't feel prepared to accept that. I tried drinking again, a few months later. A friend and I went out to a bar and a club. We had a couple of beers followed by some champagne. I thought that maybe since it was night-time, when your senses aren't quite as heightened, I might be okay. Think again, Harry: the next morning in the shower I experienced full-on panic symptoms. I knew then that I had to stop drinking. I couldn't put myself through this every time I had a swift one. I went to the doctor again, feeling a bit stupid. 'Well, Harry,' he said. 'I did say you couldn't drink …'

This time, I realised I had to take him at his word. From that day to this, I haven't touched a drop of alcohol.

Kicking the booze was good for me in so many ways: it helped to stem my anxiety and it had a hugely beneficial effect on the way I was able to do my job.

Now, I accept that my job is a bit different to most. Going on tour with the band, however, is not without its stresses and strains. Every night you're presented with the challenge of going out in front of thousands of people and putting on the best show possible. When people have paid a lot of money and looked forward to a gig for months,

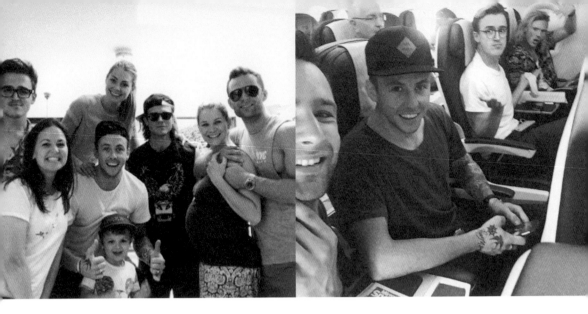

you can't have an off night or put on an average show. You're expected to relax and perform well. Over the past few years, however, I had been using alcohol to allow me to relax at gigs. I'd be hungover the next day, wake up feeling grumpy, have breakfast at midday, stagger to the tour bus and travel to the next venue. I would sometimes be pretty negative to be around and not as welcoming to the fans as I should have been. It wasn't until an hour before the next gig, when I could crack open the first beer of the day, that I would start feeling good about myself again. And so the cycle would continue.

There were times when I really hated being on stage. I'd be hungover and shaking, anxious that I wouldn't be able to get through the next song, constantly worried that I was going to mess up. I remember performing at one of the biggest arenas we'd played at in front of 15,000 people and genuinely hating the experience because I hadn't had sufficient hair of the dog before the show. It was no way to be.

AS SOON AS I QUIT THE BOOZE, ALL THAT CHANGED. I WAS MORE POSITIVE AROUND THE FANS AND A HAPPIER PERSON IN GENERAL. MY ROUTINE BECAME HEALTHIER.

My pre-show ritual became about warming up, stretching, and getting my body and mind ready for the concert. When the show was over, I found myself on a natural high from which I was able to calm down naturally, before getting a good night's sleep. I was a better performer and a better band mate, and I can remember and treasure each performance as a result.

But I wasn't totally free of on-stage anxiety.

In 2013, McFly put on four ten-year anniversary shows at the Royal Albert Hall. They were a big deal: massive gigs at perhaps the most iconic venue in the UK, if not the world. But I'd played big shows in front of big crowds at big venues before. I was completely sober. So these gigs would be fine, right?

Wrong.

There was no warning. Just a sudden realisation when I was on stage during the first night that my anxiety was unleashing itself. I started to feel the symptoms of overwhelming panic creep in. Nothing like this had ever happened on stage and the implications terrified me. I managed to get through what had become a very uncomfortable gig, but I was extremely shaky the next day and nervous about what might happen on stage that night. Thankfully I got through it and, by the time the fourth show arrived, I was able to relax a little. But I was unnerved by what had happened, not least because McFly were about to embark upon a massive new project: a collaboration with our friends from the band Busted. The forthcoming McBusted arena tour was going to be immense – by far the biggest pop tour of the year. With performances like that coming up, I knew I couldn't let this on-stage panic become a thing. I couldn't let my anxiety issues rear their ugly head while I was on stage. I had to do something about it.

It was not only my performances that I risked compromising with my anxiety. On top of everything else, I had another problem, which my anxiety exacerbated and which I had been trying to deal with over the previous few years. It was a problem that I think has been latent in me since I was young, and which has become more of an issue for me as I've grown older. That problem was obsessive-compulsive disorder, or OCD.

The idea of 'being OCD' has become a bit of a joke. You hear people saying it, light-heartedly: 'I'm a bit OCD about this or that …' And people will nod and laugh, and the conversation will carry on.

But OCD can be a serious, debilitating complaint. It has been ranked by the World Health Organization in the top ten most disabling illnesses in terms of diminished quality of life. It is an anxiety-related condition, suffered by about 12 in every 1,000 people and characterised by unwanted, unpleasant obsessions, and compulsions that need to be carried out to relieve those obsessive thoughts. I don't suppose I suffer from it to anything like the same extent as some people, but I can tell you this: it can have a substantial negative effect on the way you live your life.

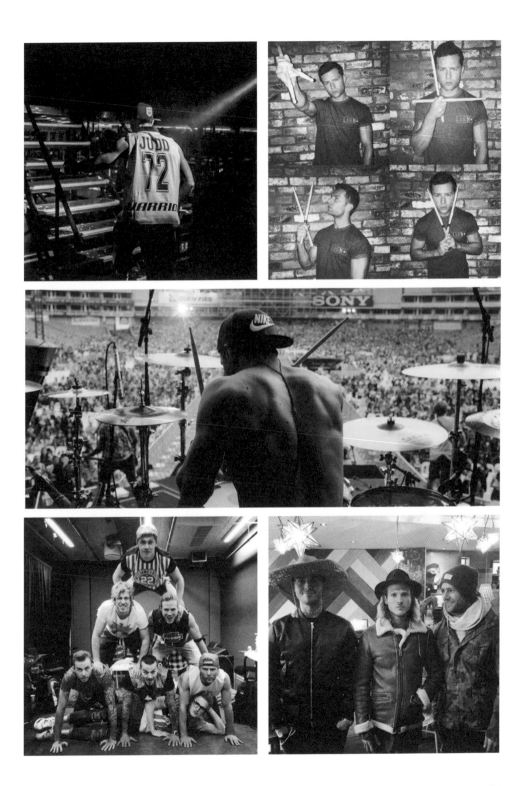

The trouble is, it can seem funny. In many instances, it *is* funny. You have my full permission to laugh at the crazy personality traits I'm about to own up to, just as I've laughed about them when I'm outside of the irrational fog of an OCD episode. When you're inside that fog, however, it can be crippling, not only for you, but also for the people around you.

If you ask my parents, they'll tell you that I displayed signs of slightly obsessive behaviour when I was a little boy. Whenever I tried to do my homework, I'd spend half the allotted time writing my name, underlining it, crossing it out, scrunching up the paper and starting it again because I wanted it to be exactly right. I'd spend ridiculous amounts of time lining up cutlery and table mats at the meal table, obsessively ensuring the angles and distances were just so. My obsessiveness really started to manifest itself, however, after I stopped smoking weed. I'd bought myself my first flat and, all of a sudden, I became totally obsessed with cleanliness and order.

It sounds funny, I know. It certainly became a joke with my friends that whenever they were around I constantly seemed to have a cleaning wipe in my hand. They laughed that I seemed to have a place for everything and showed genuine anxiety if an item was not in its place. I wanted everything to be perfect and found it difficult to cope if it wasn't. Of course, nothing ever is perfect, and when I was alone in the house, with nobody around to curb my OCD, the symptoms became far more extreme. I would find myself on all fours in my boxer shorts on the kitchen floor, sweating and obsessively cleaning every last square inch with one of my precious disinfectant wipes. In the days when I was drinking, I'd have a couple of beers with my mates and we'd howl with laughter at how ridiculous I was. The next day, though, I'd be back on my hands and knees again, scrubbing away. I couldn't relax if I knew there was a patch of limescale in the shower. When a visitor to that flat once dropped something and made a mark on the floor, I freaked out.

IT GOT TO THE POINT WHERE I COULDN'T LEAVE THE HOUSE BECAUSE I WAS OBSESSED WITH IT BEING PERFECTLY CLEAN AND HAD TO SPEND HOUR UPON HOUR MAKING IT SO.

I would feel uncontrollably anxious as I literally ran around the house, hoovering obsessively, trying to get marks off the walls and floor, and experiencing surges of anger if I couldn't.

When I moved in with Izzy – I was about 21 and we'd been together for a couple of years – my symptoms were particularly tough for her to deal with. The severity of my

OCD had been gradually increasing and, although there were no particular triggers, it was at its worst when I was at home. It was an underlying thing, always there. I remember the day we moved into our first house and the removal men scraped some furniture on the outside tiles. I went nuts: the house was ruined, we couldn't move in! It was crazy, irrational. Looking back, I find it embarrassing to admit to the way I reacted, but at the time, the frustration and anxiety seemed very real indeed.

I would stress out if Izzy invited more than a couple of people round. When she did, I would be loitering around them, trying to sneak coasters under their cups of coffee and swiping up their dirty cups to wash them and put them away before they'd even finished their drinks. On one occasion, Izzy arranged a surprise birthday party for me. I arrived home to find a whole crowd of people standing on the mezzanine area that overlooked the main room of our house. It was almost enough to give me a heart attack. While they were shouting 'Happy Birthday!', it was all I could do to stop myself yelling at them to take their shoes off! When they'd all gone, I genuinely wanted to have the flat repainted. Izzy stopped me from doing it, but I was all poised to dial the decorators …

What seems like a joke became no joke at all for her. When things were particularly bad, she couldn't relax in her own home because I couldn't relax in my own home. She felt like I was constantly watching over her, and the embarrassing truth is that I was. My OCD brought out the very worst in me. I was not only obsessive and panicky, I was starting to be nasty. If she tried to put an item down where it wasn't supposed to be, I'd be on her case. If I found a mark or a stain, I'd lose my cool, panicking that it would never come out, or that trying to get it out would make it worse. My response to any perceived imperfection in the house was completely out of proportion. I'd get it into my head that the only solution was to sell the house and start all over again. It was entirely irrational. But irrational or not, Izzy still had to deal with it.

Whenever I felt I was unable to be in control of my surroundings, I would start to feel the symptoms kick in. Autumn became my nemesis! The layout of our house meant that I had to walk through the garden in order to get out. One day I needed to be somewhere. I set out on time, but an hour later I was still in the garden, obsessively picking up leaves and twigs. It just seemed completely impossible for me to leave knowing that there was disorder in the garden. But show me a garden where there isn't disorder. We had an oak tree and a weeping willow overhanging the garden. When they dropped their leaves I would spend hours meticulously picking up every last one, even catching them as they fell, like a contestant on *The Crystal Maze*! I'd lose it if I saw another leaf fall, but it was autumn – what else were they going to do? Izzy came home one day to see that one of the bushes in our garden, which had been full of leaves when she left, was now completely bare. I had to come clean – I couldn't bear to see the leaves falling, so I'd shaken every last one off and bagged them up in a bin liner.

Ultimately, it became too much for Izzy. She had to sit me down and explain that my irrational obsessions were making it difficult for her to relax and live comfortably in her own house. I had to find some way to control my obsession. She obviously meant business and she was completely justified. This couldn't go on. It wasn't fair on Izzy and, when our daughter Lola came along, it wasn't fair on her either. I didn't want my wife and daughter to see this irrational, angry side of my nature. I had to do something to get on top of it.

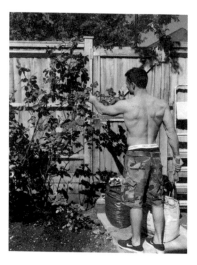

ANXIETY. PANIC ATTACKS. OCD. I WAS BEGINNING TO TICK OFF QUITE A CHECKLIST OF MENTAL HEALTH ISSUES!

Gradually, I became accustomed to the idea that I was just going to have to be careful with myself. I needed to sleep well – to go to bed at a reasonable hour and get myself seven or eight hours a night. I needed to eat well, because I knew that on days when I filled myself with rubbish food and gorged on sugar, I could start to feel pretty uncomfortable.

But most of all, I needed to do the one thing that, as I will explain in the next chapter, over the years had become my constant, my stress-reliever, my escape from anxiety and my release. The one thing that kept my OCD at bay. The one thing that I knew had the power to get my head in the right place and keep it there.

I needed to exercise.

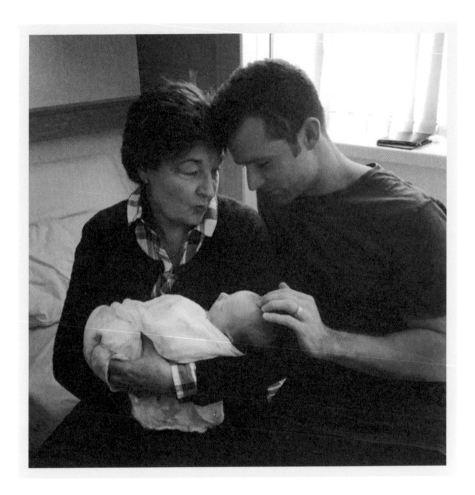

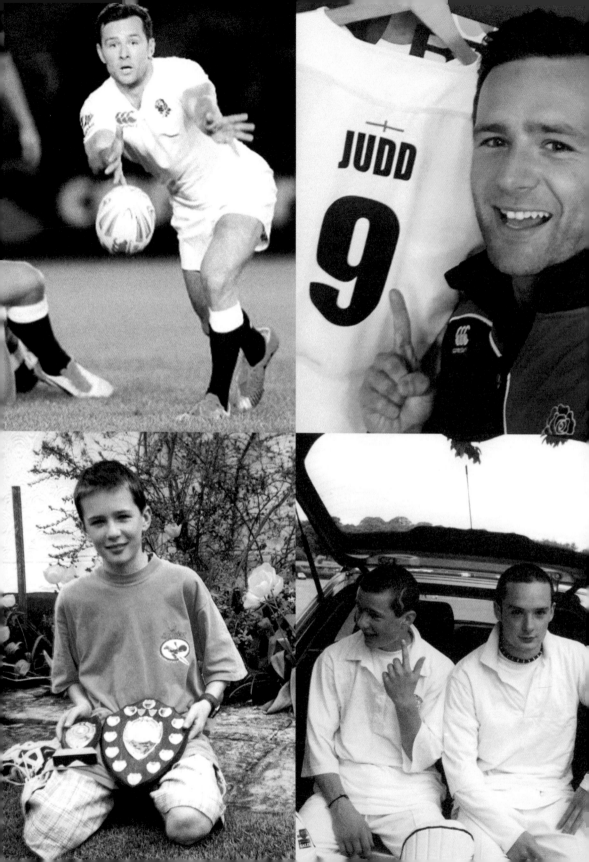

GET FIT, GET HAPPY

When I was a kid and a teenager, in the days before McFly and everything that went with being in a successful band, sport was a big part of my life.

Now, I believe sport and exercise are not the same thing, for reasons that I hope will become clear. However, growing up, sport was a huge thing for me: my gateway drug, if you like, to the world of physical activity and all the benefits it has to offer.

As a kid, I turned my hand to pretty much any sport I could – football, tennis, rugby, hockey, you name it. I was successful on the sports field. I made the first teams in every sport at school. When I was 12 and at boarding school in Suffolk, a friend and I used to while away the long winter nights playing table tennis. We became pretty good, winning the Suffolk championship with our four-man school team, then the East Anglian championship, and eventually coming second in the South of England championship. We proudly announced to our school friends that this put us third in the country, since the South of England went on to beat the North of England. Whether that was true or not, I don't know, but it was certainly an early taste of the euphoria that playing a bit of sport with other people can give you!

My real love, though, was cricket. I was captain of the school team and played some childhood county cricket for Suffolk. When I was 11, my mum took me down to Lord's Indoor Cricket School for their Easter course. While I was there, the guys from the Marylebone Cricket Club (MCC) spotted me and I was asked to come and do a trial for their School of Merit (they sometimes referred to it as the School of Excellence, which I rather preferred!). There was a big board at the indoor school with a list of cricketers who'd passed through the School of Merit: I was star-struck seeing names like Mike Atherton and Graham Gooch up there, and thinking that maybe I had a chance of being one of them. I did the trial and had a full-on Billy Elliot moment in my bedroom when the result letter arrived. I was convinced I wouldn't be accepted, but I was. It was a big moment in my young life.

Every third weekend I travelled down to London for a couple of days' training, surrounded by all these brilliant young cricketers aged between 11 and 13. It fired me up, being in this elite programme where I could play with some of the best kids in the country. My prep school was happy for me to go down to London to do this, but when I moved to my senior school they were less keen, so I had to give it up. I wasn't too upset: the standard of cricket at my new school was high, and my passion for it was undiminished.

There was a lot of expectation on me as a cricketer when I moved to my senior school. Here I was, a new boy who'd been spotted by the MCC and who was supposedly a bit special. In my first year, I completely failed to live up to that expectation. I buckled under the pressure. I bombed. It was the worst season of my life. My highest score was about 26 and I don't think I hit a single boundary. It was very different from my performances at prep school, where I'd been captain of cricket and had won the competition that awarded points for the most runs and most wickets. Suddenly my confidence had deserted me, and I was awful.

Things turned around in my second year. I scored a couple of fifties, and gradually my confidence started to return. I remember thinking that after two decent games, it didn't much matter what I did for the rest of the season. The shackles were off and, now that I wasn't worrying about my performance, I started to show what I could do. I got myself a school record when I scored 163 not out against Bedford School, out of a team score of 199. Next game, I topped even that, scoring 179 not out. I was moved up to the school First XI, playing with the under-18s and performing well for them. I scored a couple of half-centuries and was even awarded my school colours. Bear in mind that this was a pretty posh school. Earning your colours gave you the right to wear a white cap, a white blazer and – wait for it – a special cravat! It was the proudest moment of my life, walking round school in that cravat. Never mind that they didn't make the white blazers in my tiny, prepubescent size – I didn't start growing until I was 15. It was enormous on me and I can only think that I must have looked ridiculous.

But I loved my cricket. That summer I played for my club, scored a couple of centuries for them and even played for the men's team. I felt unstoppable. I was genuinely thinking that I wanted to take it to the next level: to go up to county level and see where that road might lead me. If I'm being entirely honest with myself, I doubt that I was really good enough to become a professional player, but cricket was certainly the most important activity in my life at that time.

The following Easter, however, disaster struck. I contracted glandular fever. I had to spend a lot more time at home, so my presence at school was sporadic. When the cricket term came around, I had a pretty average season, largely because I was in and out of school (though somehow I did manage to blag missing lessons while being allowed to play cricket!). My cricketing career had peaked. My glory days at the crease were over. I was still in the cricket team, but I remember going to Bedford School again and seeing a young cricketer who was scoring double centuries for fun, and realising that I wasn't at that level – I don't mind though, he was none other than former England captain, Alastair Cook, after all.

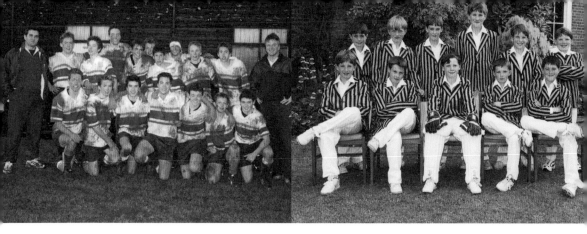

My schoolboy cricketing career had had its ups and downs. But although I probably didn't realise it at the time, I think I learned an important lesson about sport in general: confidence is everything. When I was confident, I was riding high; when I lacked confidence, not so much. I suggested at the beginning of this chapter that sport and exercise are not the same thing. For me, this is perhaps the biggest difference between the two. We sometimes lack confidence in sport because we worry about our results. When my scores on the cricket pitch were low, I felt I was somehow failing. It may sound silly but it was everything to me and when I wasn't performing well it hit me hard. It's the same with other aspects of my life too – the anxiety really came out. This is not the case with exercise.

AT THE CORE OF MY PHILOSOPHY IS ONE SIMPLE TRUTH: YOU CAN'T FAIL AT EXERCISE. YOU CAN'T BE BAD AT IT.

You either do it, or you don't. It's important that you remember this as you read the pages that follow. I'm not here to force you to compete, or to set you up to fail. There will be no First XIs, no cricketing colours and no posh cravats.

Once I was back at school full-time, I continued to play cricket and other sports. And although I carried on in all the first teams, I was no longer the boy wonder I briefly appeared to be. Perhaps that was a good thing. Perhaps I was learning that the real benefits of taking part in sporting activities are less to do with competition and more to

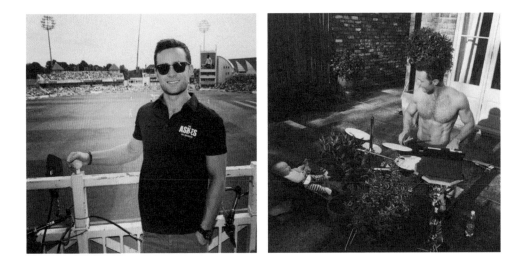

do with keeping active, getting outside in the fresh air and feeling like you're part of a team. Before long, however, my love of sport was joined by a new enthusiasm: I started playing the drums. I used to tell everyone that I wanted to be a cricketer or a drummer. In the privacy of my own thoughts, however, I felt I wasn't really good enough to do either professionally, no matter how much I might enjoy them.

Thankfully, the drumming thing worked out. But when I joined McFly, all my sporting activity went out of the window as I became a full-on, bona fide stoner for two years. It was a few years later that my interest in sport returned.

When I was 21, I was asked by a family friend to play in a charity cricket match in Cambridge in aid of the Teenage Cancer Trust. It was a cause that I felt close to, since a friend of mine had battled cancer while he was a teenager. I was to be on a team of locals and teenage cancer patients, against a celebrity team called the Bunburys. Run by a real character called David English, the Bunburys comprise lots of former cricketers. When I went out to bat and scored – to everyone's surprise – 75 not out, David English was all over me. He extravagantly dubbed me 'the right-handed David Gower' and roped me into playing for the team. I did so for the next few years. It was quite an experience for a cricket enthusiast, as I got to play with so many of my childhood heroes: Darren Gough, Phil Tufnell, Mark Ramprakash, Freddie Flintoff and Devon Malcolm, to name a few. Playing for Ian Botham's eleven, I had a great partnership with Kevin Pietersen's brother Bryan (85 not out, and I hit Darren Gough for a six – if you don't believe me, ask him!), and I even began to recover some of my old form, scoring 110 (not out!) against Craig White, who had bowled the fastest ever ball recorded by an English fast bowler. (Have you noticed by now that I'm pretty good at remembering my cricket scores? I'm also pretty good at showing off – if you don't back yourself, no one else will!)

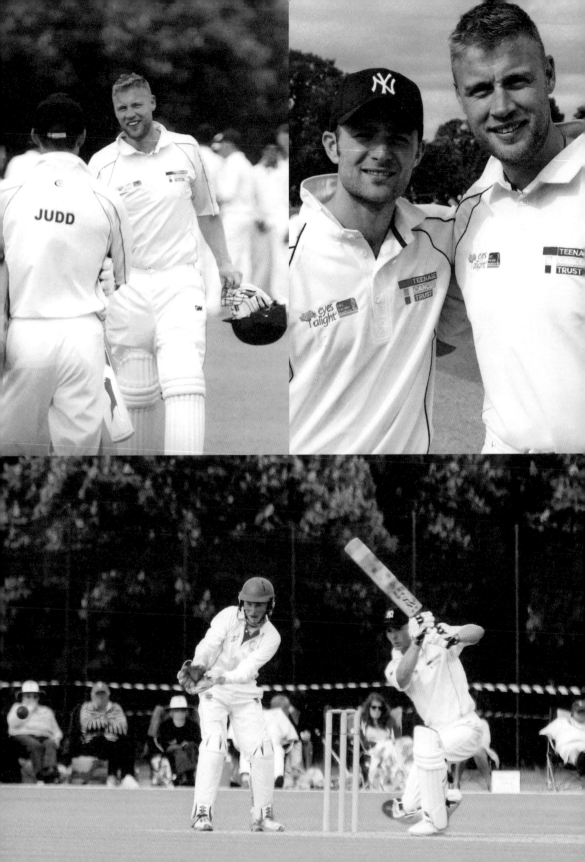

More importantly, however, after spending two years doing the most destructive, unproductive thing I could possibly do, this felt like a step in the right direction with respect to my health and general well-being. I felt better in myself for getting out there and being active, and was beginning to understand that the benefits of exercise could be more far-reaching than I'd previously realised. This understanding was consolidated when, in 2006, I travelled to India on behalf of Sport Relief, along with a contingent of sportsmen and other personalities: Phil Tufnell, Andy Flower, Chris Evans, Dermot O'Leary, Jake Humphrey, and lots of others.

This was not the first time I'd travelled to a disadvantaged part of the world. In January 2005, McFly had travelled to Uganda for Comic Relief, a heart-wrenching, traumatic trip that left us all feeling humbled by the hardships some people have to endure, and very grateful for what we had. In some respects, India was similar. The Sport Relief trip happened just after the tsunami had struck. Our intention was to make a film to raise awareness of the plight of these poor people whose homes had been destroyed and whose families had been torn apart. It was heartbreaking stuff.

We were there, however, to show how sport can have a positive effect in even the most desperate scenarios such as this. A cricket match was organised: us against a team of locals, on a strip of grass by the beach. Hundreds of local Indian kids came to watch and the atmosphere was absolutely incredible. I kept wicket and went out to bat. While I was playing, the local kids started to chant 'Dhoni! Dhoni!', after the Indian player who was also a wicketkeeper and batsman.

It became clear to me that day just how much the sport meant to the people of India. Even in the midst of their terrible predicament after the tsunami, the sight of a bunch of English guys coming out and simply having a game with them was evidently a positive experience. I certainly don't want to be trite and suggest in any way that a game of cricket was the cure for all of their problems, but I left India reminded that sport has a singular power, even in the most difficult situations and for just a brief moment, to make things seem better.

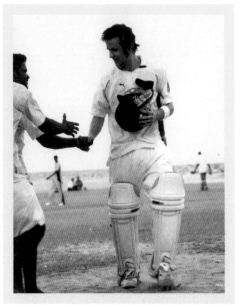

It was a thought that would go on to have a great resonance in my own life.

It felt good to be involved in physical activity again. It was a welcome distraction from my bouts of anxiety and OCD. Of course, I was still drinking and smoking tobacco back in 2006 so it could hardly be said that I was a picture of physical health. Having struck up a relationship with the Teenage Cancer Trust, however, I felt I wanted to do something to raise awareness and funds for them. I decided to run the London Marathon on their behalf in April 2008.

Getting up to match fitness for a marathon was a big ask. Happily, I found the ideal place to do it. In January 2008 the band headed to Australia for ten weeks to work on the music that would become the album *Radio:Active*. We were looking forward to partying, and the partying started with a pretty intense session on the beers immediately when we arrived. It was a grey cold day, we were jet-lagged and we woke up the following morning feeling pretty terrible, but greeted by some incredible weather. From that moment, we were inspired to find our kicks elsewhere.

We started surfing every day. Something about the fresh air, the salt water and the exercise had an amazingly inspiring effect on all four of us.

WE SUDDENLY WEREN'T INTERESTED IN PARTYING IN THE WAY THAT WE THOUGHT WE WOULD BE. WE JUST WANTED TO CATCH THE WAVES REGULARLY AND EAT HEALTHILY.

We were more interested in smoothies than beers! We were really tapping into the healthy Australian lifestyle. We felt completely buzzed, the band spirit was great and we were hugely productive in the studio. We were having the time of our lives, and I personally think it was all down to physical activity and healthy living. The vibe was awesome.

I'd asked lots of people to sponsor me for the marathon, but I was feeling a bit of a fraud because to date I'd done nothing to get in shape for that April. I was in the perfect place to rectify that, however. I didn't have to look too far before I found someone who could help me. There was a guy doing training sessions with members of the public on the beach. I approached him, explained that I was from England and that I was running a marathon. Could he help me get ready for it?

He sure could. We started training on the beach. Despite all my cricket, this was the first major bit of exercise I'd done since being at school. It was incredible. I got such a buzz from it, such a high. It was a reminder of the person I used to be before all my physical and mental health problems got in the way. This, combined with all the positives of being in Australia with the guys, meant I found myself in a very happy place.

I completed the marathon in April. And while my smoking and drinking certainly held me back to a certain extent, I can honestly say that the marathon gave me the biggest adrenaline rush I've ever experienced – and that includes getting to number one in the charts and playing to packed-out crowds at Wembley. It was a genuine high point of my life.

Sometimes, when you try to recreate a moment, it doesn't work. In 2010 we returned to Australia, hoping to recapture the vibe of our first trip. It didn't happen, and I feel that I shoulder some of the responsibility for that. I was going through a bout of anxiety and being away from home seemed to make it worse.

We arrived in Australia and I was a mess again. Crippled by anxiety, I was unable to break out of it. I couldn't bring myself to do anything. When people tell me that they find it difficult to motivate themselves to get active when they're feeling low, I remember that second trip to Australia and I really do understand what they mean. I surfed maybe once and my state of mind got in the way of being able to take advantage of the weather, the outdoor lifestyle, the whole Australian vibe. I was anxious 24/7, and I think it had an effect on the guys. Nothing really happened in the studio. Our attempt to recreate what we had before simply failed. I accept a large proportion of the blame for that. I was in an absolute state.

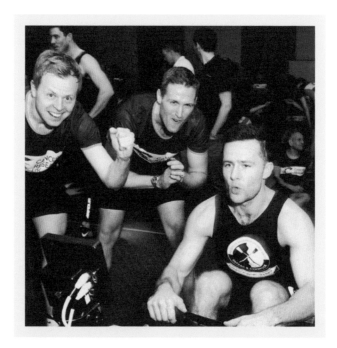

The episode passed. Around 2010, we decided as a band that we needed to stop looking so scruffy and unhealthy and do something to get into shape. Maybe it's my addictive personality, or my competitiveness, but I took this decision pretty seriously. I found myself a personal trainer and started hitting the gym regularly. Initially my working out was purely aesthetic and it soon started to have the desired effect on the way I looked but I wasn't yet aware of the other benefits exercise would bring. But I still, slightly, felt like a bit of a fraud. I was doing weight training and I was an ambassador for the Teenage Cancer Trust, but I was still a smoker.

Smoking is ridiculous. We all know that. But I do sympathise with smokers. I took a year psyching myself up to stop. What got me over the line was, undoubtedly, exercise.

Smoking was particularly stupid for me. I only started at 15 to try and look cool, but as well as being physically just about the most unhealthy vice, it also brought on my anxiety. Every day became a constant battle as I tried not to smoke too much. Each morning I would put off my first cigarette because I knew it would induce my anxiety – which I find is always worse in the morning anyway. When I failed, as I inevitably would, I'd get annoyed with myself. I was a smoker who didn't want to be a smoker, but I was hooked and couldn't let it go. I didn't know how to tackle it. And in some ways I suppose I was conflicted. The thought of giving up cigarettes made me freak out! I'd quit weed, I'd quit booze … smoking was my final vice, the last bit of rebel still inside me. Part of me wanted to quit, part of me wanted to stay the same. And if I couldn't have a cigarette, what would I do with myself when I went to the pub and all my mates were standing outside smoking?

I stood at this crossroads for a year, maybe more, battling with myself every day. Then, on New Year's Eve 2012, I went to the pub with some friends near Izzy's mum and dad's house. No longer being a drinker, I smoked my way through the entire evening and into the small hours. We got back to Izzy's parents' house at about four in the morning. Izzy herself had quit smoking in 2008. Exhausted, she said she was going to bed. I told her I'd be up in a minute, once I'd had one last cigarette.

I went outside. I stank of tobacco. I'd smoked so much that evening that my chest was hurting. Halfway through my cigarette, I looked at the smouldering tube between my fingers and thought: this is disgusting. I was so fed up with it. I put the cigarette out and flicked the stub into the bushes. I remember thinking to myself (though not really believing it): I wonder if that's going to be the last cigarette I ever smoke. It was.

I woke up the next morning with a sudden determination in my head. I was going to give up smoking.

Izzy and I travelled to my parents' house that day and I grandly announced in front of them that I was quitting. They were as pleased to hear it as I was to have made the decision. Within hours, however, the high of telling people I'd quit had worn off. And the craving had kicked in.

It was about half past four in the afternoon. My brother, also a smoker, was rolling himself a cigarette, and I was already on the verge of cracking, my willpower crumbling with each second that passed. I hadn't even quit for 24 hours and already I couldn't hack it. No.

I WASN'T GOING TO GIVE IN. I DECIDED THAT INSTEAD OF SMOKING A CIGARETTE, I'D PUT ON MY TRAINERS AND GO FOR A RUN.

It was pitch-black outside and freezing. After half a mile, as the cold air hit my damaged smoker's lungs, my chest was in agony. I fought through it and pounded out two or three miles. Physically it was very uncomfortable – I couldn't help wondering what harm I'd done myself with all the smoking – but mentally I was feeling incredibly positive. I decided I had to take it just one day at a time and told myself that I would smoke again so it felt like less of a mountain to climb. Knowing that I could stop trying to quit definitely helped me but I never did. The exercise gave me an incredible sense of elation. The cigarette craving had gone, the endorphins were pumping round my body and all I could think about was getting out there again tomorrow to continue the process of repairing all the damage I'd been doing to myself. (And when I went to bed that night and Izzy told me how much nicer it was that I didn't smell of smoke, I can't deny it was an extra incentive.)

I'M NOT HERE TO TELL YOU THAT QUITTING SMOKING WAS EASY. IT CERTAINLY WASN'T. WITHOUT QUESTION, HOWEVER, THE GREATEST WEAPON IN MY ARSENAL WAS EXERCISE.

Whenever the urge to smoke threatened to become overwhelming, I got outside and went for a run. And every time I ran, I experienced the same high I'd had that New Year's Day. In a sense, I was replacing one high with another, but there was no doubt in my mind that the exercise high was one hell of a sight better for me than any of the highs I'd experienced to date. Exercise was, slowly but surely, changing my life.

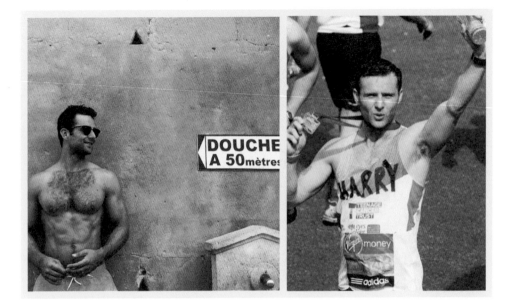

Maybe I took it to too much of an extreme. I was going to run a second London Marathon in April 2013. This time, my training was far more vigorous than first time round. Free of the shackles of my smoking addiction, I went at it full pelt. I did one long run a week, two lots of interval training (alternating periods of high- and low-intensity exercise), strength training, hill sprints … you name it. I took it to another level and perhaps pushed myself too hard. A month or so before the race, I felt what I thought was a twitch in my left pectoral muscle. I ignored it for a week or so, but when I mentioned it to Izzy, she packed me off straight away to a cardiologist. I got wired up and underwent a bunch of tests, before being diagnosed with a condition called a 'wandering pacemaker'. The cardiologist explained that sometimes, when you become very fit and your resting heart rate becomes very low, your heart acts as its own pacemaker to keep itself going. It often happens with athletes and isn't harmful. I was fine to run the marathon, but should maybe calm down on the interval training. I took his advice, put more of an emphasis on strength-based training and the condition went away on its own. Nowadays, I still do some interval training, but I've never pushed myself quite that hard since. Izzy doesn't want me to do any more marathons – she can't cope with me and my obsessive training! I will, though. It's the best feeling ever. To anyone thinking about it, I can't recommend the experience highly enough. I can honestly say finishing the marathon (twice) was one of the biggest adrenaline rushes I've experienced. There was a point in the race both times when my body and mind were ready to give in but it felt like someone had injected me with a shot of adrenaline and all the pain disappeared. It felt like I was floating as I crossed the finish line.

Gradually, over a period of more than ten years, exercise had found its way into my life. It had taught me so much. In India I had seen the power of sport to bring people together and help, in some small way, those who had suffered terrible hardship. While running the marathon I had seen how people could come together through exercise to raise money and achieve positive results for those suffering a huge range of awful illnesses. And I'd used it to raise awareness and funds for charities close to my own heart, such as the Teenage Cancer Trust and the Brain Injury Rehabilitation Trust (which Izzy and I support because Izzy's brother Rupert suffered a brain injury in a terrible car crash).

But there was more to it than that. It's no exaggeration to say that exercise has helped me turn my life around. It had been my go-to weapon in the battle to stop smoking. It had helped fill the gap left when I stopped drinking alcohol. And it had massively improved my ability to do my job as a musician. Take rehearsals, for instance. Rehearsing for a big show is a busy time: you're learning a lot and making demands on your body as you play. In the old days, I would sit on the Tube or in a taxi on the way to rehearsals and arrived feeling lethargic and grumpy. I'd be ducking out at every opportunity for a cigarette break. It used to be a band joke that Harry was yawning his way through rehearsals! Now, whenever I can, I cycle – my version of commuting to work. I arrive feeling energised and positive, buzzing and productive. I can't wait to get started and I enjoy playing the drums so much more. I also enjoy touring more. Those days blighted by alcohol and physical inactivity are far behind me. Now I'm up early, exercising and living right. I'm more focused, but crucially I'm happier. Exercise has made a profound difference to my life as a band member and my happiness in the band.

Most importantly, I have found that

WHENEVER THE SYMPTOMS OF ANXIETY OR OCD ENCROACH ON MY LIFE, I CAN BEAT THEM BACK WITH JUST A LITTLE EXERCISE.

The more active I am, the less I find myself to be in the grip of these strange compulsions.

I can't overstate how much exercise has changed me for the better. I have come to accept that anxiety and OCD are issues that will probably be with me for the rest of my life. I can't pretend that I'm completely relaxed around the house. I can't pretend that I'm not forever sorting my clothes or lining up my shoes. I can't pretend that my Dyson vacuum cleaner doesn't need replacing yearly, I use it so much. If I have time

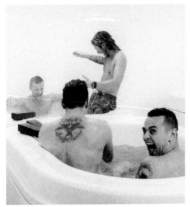
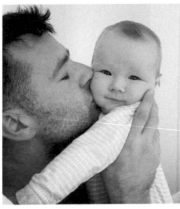
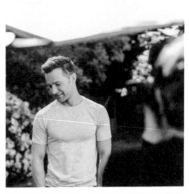
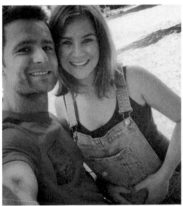
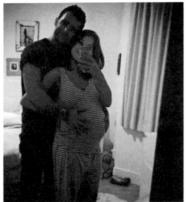
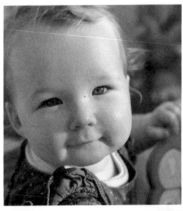
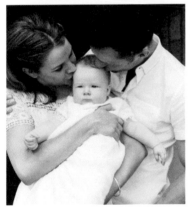
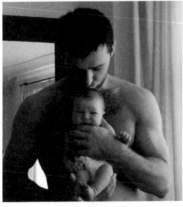
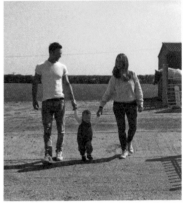
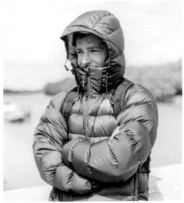
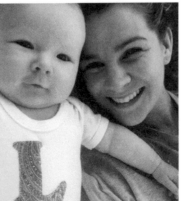
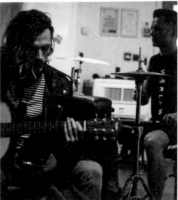

on my hands, chances are I'll be stalking round the house in my boxers, sandpaper in one hand, silicone gun in the other, as I rectify certain imperfections only I can see. But I can leave the house knowing there's a bit of tidying up to do. I can let someone drink a cup of coffee without swiping it away from them (this is no exaggeration, I go into auto-pilot and start clearing things away – I've often been asked by guests where their cup of coffee has gone when they were only halfway through!). And I can accept that it's autumn and there are going to be leaves!

Slowly but surely, I am learning. In Lola's room there is an upholstered chair. Some months ago, we spilt some milk on it. I completely lost it. Now, the stains on that chair are a constant test to me. As I write these words, just a few hours ago I entered the room to see a fresh stain on the chair. My initial response was one of panic, but I managed to tell myself – and crucially to believe – that it really didn't matter. This is real progress for me!

That progress has exercise at its core and I'm not the only one in the Judd household who benefits from it. As I was writing this, Izzy reminded me of her own difficulties with anxiety – different to mine, but no less consequential. It's amazing how it held her back as a professional violinist. She found that travelling and being away from home would trigger her own anxiety, which had held her back from pursuing the life of a performer. Her anxiety has been part of my life just as mine has been part of hers. In fact, there were times when it started to have quite a detrimental effect on our relationship. As she's grown as a person and learned how to deal with it in the same way that I have, exercise has become a vital part of her routine.

We each take time to ourselves to exercise. Different couples will find different ways of managing it. Later in the book you'll see some workouts specially designed for couples to do together (see pages 104–111). I truly believe that building exercise into your relationship is important and mutually beneficial, even if that is just taking time to go for a walk together. It can have a positive effect on so many different parts of your life. When Izzy and I had difficulties conceiving, it led to long periods of terrible frustration for us. After a couple of years of this, Izzy found the need to completely reset herself. She focused 100 per cent on her own health and well-being. When Izzy exercised I could see how it made her more positive and I was confident, along with yoga and eating well helped. It made her feel more positive about our situation to know that she was doing everything she could that was within her control.

Small wonder, then, that I am passionate about making this part of our own family life, and that our children should see exercise as being a natural, ordinary, regular part of their day. I've even set Lola up in her baby bouncer before now and done a half-hour workout while she bobs up and down watching me. When our children are older, I hope we'll keep fit together, because I know how much it has benefited both Izzy and me. I'm certain it will be a positive way of spending time together and focusing on each other, away from screens and the other distractions of modern life.

Every day I am aware of the need to take care of myself. If I don't, the demons banging on the door might find a way in. I'm still prone to anxiety, particularly in the morning and especially if I've had a busy few days and I fail to eat properly, sleep properly or have enough exercise. I wake up with the familiar burning knot in my stomach.

Only now, I have a strategy to deal with it. I get moving. Perhaps I'll go for a run. Perhaps I'll do a workout in my living room. Perhaps I'll go to the gym. It doesn't need to be much – sometimes it's just for five to ten minutes – but the effects are almost magical. After a bit of exercise, everything seems better. I can face the day. I can see my irrational thoughts for what they are. I can be productive. If I exercise in the morning, I'm tired enough to sleep properly come evening. The cycle is broken and I'm back where I should be. It's my form of meditation: a way of shutting off and being in the moment. It's also something that I can control.

This, then, is why I'm passionate about exercise. It's not just to do with the aesthetic benefits of working out – they're simply a bonus. For me, the real reason to exercise is that it makes me feel good.

Long story short: exercise keeps me, and my family, in a happier place.

The positive effect exercise was having on my mood was so profound, so life-changing, that I started to become evangelical about it! I wanted to spread the word. I felt confident that the symptoms of anxiety and OCD that I was experiencing were extremely common in guys and girls, young and old. And even people who don't have these disorders also now and then succumb to the stresses and strains of modern life. We all have moments when our mood could do with a boost. We all have our ups and downs and times when we feel blue.

With this in mind, I began to think that maybe I could help people get the same benefits from exercise that I've enjoyed. I was very conscious that I didn't want to be preachy – I know people don't like being told what to do, especially by a drummer in a pop band who likes to dance on the telly and pose nude on the front of magazines! I wanted to come up with a different approach. First, though, I needed to get my facts straight. I wanted to find out as much as I could about the positive health benefits – both mental and physical – of exercise, from the people who really know about the subject.

It was time to speak to some experts. I decided to go on a fact-finding mission.

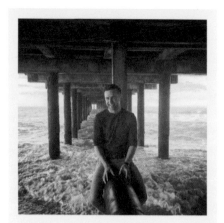

THE MIRACLE PILL

Anyone who has ever suffered from any kind of mental health issue, be it anxiety, OCD, depression or something else, will have been told that exercise can, in many cases, be as effective as medication or talking therapies when it comes to overcoming these debilitating conditions. Now, don't get me wrong. I understand how difficult this can be. Sometimes, when my anxiety's at its worst, it can be tough even to get out of the house, let alone exercise. But while I'm not suggesting that exercise is a cure-all, I definitely wanted to find out more about how it can make a difference to people's mood.

It was clear to me from my own experience, that the positive mental health benefits of exercise go hand in hand with so many other health benefits that it can be hard to separate them. Our minds and our bodies are part of the same entity. It seemed to me that before I could understand why exercise is good for your head, I needed to understand why it is good for your body.

I decided to hunt down an expert in the subject. So I found myself sitting down with the incredibly knowledgeable Professor Sanjay Sharma, Professor of Cardiology at St George's, University of London. Professor Sharma is the guy. He is the consultant cardiologist for the charitable organisation Cardiac Risk in the Young, and Lead for the Inherited Cardiomyopathies and Sports Cardiology Unit at St George's. His interests include studying the hearts of sportsmen, and his particular field of research is activities and interventions that can either improve the functioning of the heart or, more extremely, that might be harmful for a sportsperson, even to the extent of killing them. He has spent a substantial part of his career looking after the best hearts in the country – hearts belonging to sportsmen such as Jonny Wilkinson and Mo Farah. He has also looked after some of the worst hearts, belonging to young people with very serious heart diseases. He knows his stuff.

Professor Sharma explained to me in very simple terms how good exercise is for our bodies. People who exercise regularly, he told me, are less likely to be overweight, they are more likely to have better blood pressure and cholesterol results than people who don't exercise, and they are less likely to have diabetes. He explained that

BY CONTROLLING METRICS SUCH AS OBESITY, BLOOD PRESSURE AND DIABETES, WE CAN REDUCE OUR RISK OF HEART ATTACKS WHEN WE'RE IN OUR FIFTIES AND SIXTIES BY AS MUCH AS 50 PER CENT.

That sounded like an astonishing statistic to me, but Professor Sharma went further.

ON AVERAGE, HE TOLD ME, PEOPLE WHO EXERCISE LIVE ABOUT SEVEN YEARS LONGER THAN PEOPLE WHO DON'T EXERCISE AT ALL.

Who wouldn't want that? That is more time to exercise! This is not just because of the benefits of exercise to the heart, but also because exercise can prevent certain cancers, notably of the prostate, the breast and the colon. Exercise is anti-ageing – it improves your cognition, your concentration, your confidence and your stamina levels. And not only can exercise give us a *longer* life, it can give us a *better* life. It is an antidepressant and it almost certainly slows the onset of dementia.

IF YOU PACKAGED EXERCISE INTO A TABLET, PROFESSOR SHARMA TOLD ME, IT WOULD BE KNOWN AS 'THE MIRACLE PILL'.

The miracle pill. That was a phrase that really resonated with me. I had started exercising because I enjoyed it and it made me feel great. I knew it was 'good' for you, but I wanted validation from some professionals. I was even more taken aback when Professor Sharma told me how detrimental to health physical inactivity can be. We know, he explained, that people who don't exercise at all are more likely to be overweight, more likely to be depressed and much more likely to have all the risk factors – such as high blood pressure, high cholesterol and diabetes – that you require to end up with a heart attack in later life.

PHYSICAL INACTIVITY, HE TOLD ME, IS THE NEW SMOKING.

Clearly, that's a big problem. But our response to it is not the same as our response to the dangers of smoking. Professor Sharma made the point that every single health professional spends their life telling people not to smoke. Not so with exercise. Think about it … how often do you hear it talked about? He takes the view that, before reaching for the prescription pad and handing out a tablet that will make someone feel better, every single medical consultation should end with some advice about how good exercise is. He believes that health professionals should focus on preventing disease as much as curing it. He takes the view that, if people heeded this advice, the 120,000 deaths from heart attacks that we see in the UK each year could be reduced by about 40 per cent.

Professor Sharma made another point that resonated with me because it echoed my own experience: that exercise promotes healthy living in other respects. If you're committed to exercise and you've decided to go out and have a run at seven o'clock in the morning, you're less likely to stay up late and do those things you're going to regret in the morning. If you're in a team, you're more likely to adopt a healthier lifestyle. Chances are your diet will change because you don't want to undo all your good work by eating junk food. If you're a smoker, perhaps you'll stop.

All these were true for me. Although I try not to be too obsessive about my diet, it's undoubtedly true that I eat cleaner, healthier food now that I'm exercising. I've cut down on the sugar and junk food, in favour of healthier options. And, nutrition aside, exercise has been the catalyst for so many good decisions I've made in my life, such as quitting smoking and alcohol, concentrating on sleeping better and enjoying work more. Professor Sharma was confirming that this is generally the case.

I was interested to know the professor's opinions on why, since the benefits of exercise are so clear, people still struggle to make it a priority in their lives. He put it largely down to education. In his opinion, every GP's surgery should carry a poster shouting about the benefits of exercise. More than that, he felt that we should be promoting exercise on TV, advertising it in the same way that we advertise butter or cream. We should be talking about exercise on radio shows or even at gigs – making all the benefits it bestows cool, rather than a drag. That made a lot of sense to me and it chimed strongly with my own desire to get the word out about how exercise has massively improved my own life.

Professor Sharma was equally clear about the responsibilities held by parents and schools. He observed that there is very little talk in our school curriculum about physical activity and its positive impact on health. Many schools have stopped doing PE altogether, which was compulsory not so many years ago. This is a problem, because if you're fit as a youngster, you'll find it much easier to get fit when you go back to exercise as an adult.

I found this particularly interesting because, as a new father, I have one simple hope for my daughter. For as long as I can remember, the importance of eating healthy food has been drilled into us. Everybody knows that we should eat our five a day, that we should lay off the fizzy drinks, sweets and crisps and try not to fill ourselves up with sugar. Exercise is just as important, yet we have few guidelines that all of us have instinctively learned. When it comes to exercise and children, how often do we simply hear people say, 'Get them outside for a bit so they sleep tonight'? It's unfocused and half-hearted.

MY AIM IS TO BE ABLE TO SAY TO MY DAUGHTER, 'LET'S GO OUTSIDE AND DO OUR DAILY TEN MINUTES.'

I want it to become just as much a part of our daily routine as brushing our teeth. As I was learning, exercise has so many benefits, in so many ways, that I'd feel remiss if I didn't help my daughter build an awareness of it into her life, just as I know she'll grow up with an awareness of the importance of good nutrition.

Of course, even when people understand the benefits of exercise, it's often the case that they still don't put that knowledge into action. I have long been interested to know why. In my own research, I commonly encounter four recurring excuses that people give whenever I ask them why they are not physically active. These four excuses are: they don't have the time, they don't have the money, they don't have the motivation and they feel intimidated by going to the gym. I'm determined to find a way of breaking down these four obstacles. I hope to show that exercise doesn't have to take up a load of your time, that it doesn't have to cost anything, that motivation is just a matter of being a little bit creative and there's really nothing to feel intimidated about. A plan was starting to form in my mind.

Professor Sharma seemed to agree. He was quite adamant that it isn't really true that exercise has to take up a huge chunk of your time. On the contrary,

'THE AMOUNT OF EXERCISE NEEDED TO GET THE FULL HEALTH BENEFITS THAT HE HAD OUTLINED — THE LONGER LIFE, THE STRONGER HEART, THE IMPROVED WELL-BEING AND GENERAL HEALTH — WERE RELATIVELY MODEST.'

He suggested that walking briskly, or jogging, for no more than two hours in a whole week, divided into three or four sessions, would be sufficient.

He was quite clear about two things in this respect. Firstly, that a good proportion of that exercise could be achieved through small lifestyle changes. For example, instead of taking a car or a bus from A to B: walk. Instead of standing on the escalator every day: climb. Instead of taking the lift: use the stairs. Small bursts of activity like this soon add up, and in this way it doesn't take much for us to achieve the optimal levels of exercise. By building these techniques into your day, you don't have to take so much time out of it for dedicated exercise.

Secondly, any sort of exercise is better than none at all. Clearly we're not all able to devote massive amounts of time to the business of keeping fit, or exercise to the same level as Premier League footballers or professional long-distance runners. Some of us might even have ailments that make it more difficult for us to get active to the extent that Professor Sharma was suggesting – neurological disease, perhaps, or arthritis. But we should not think that just because we can't reach the 'recommended' levels of exercise, we should give up on it completely. Even a small amount of exercise can make a big difference. He laid another amazing statistic on me:

IF YOU GO RUNNING FOR AN HOUR A WEEK, YOU REDUCE YOUR CHANCE OF A HEART ATTACK BY 48 PER CENT. NOT A BAD RETURN ON YOUR TIME INVESTMENT.

Running like that might not be possible for everyone but every bit of exercise has a positive impact.

What about the expense of exercise? Well, you can take a brisk walk anywhere. It certainly doesn't require an expensive gym membership and you don't need exercise machines to go for a run. You don't even need weights to do weight training: a lot of very well-built people don't use weights at all, but exercise using their own body weight.

And as for motivation, it's just a question of choosing the right type of exercise and maybe thinking outside the box a little. I totally get that people might find the idea of relentless weightlifting off-putting. I completely understand that, for some, the thought of sweating it out on the cross trainer or rowing machine, or of pounding the pavements in your running shoes, is a complete turn-off. But physical activity doesn't have to be any of those things. It can be a kick-around in the park. It can be a romantic walk in the woods. Most of all it was becoming clearer that it needed to be *fun*.

IT COULD EVEN BE 20 MINUTES ENERGETICALLY DANCING TO YOUR FAVOURITE ALBUM.

All these alternative activities, and more, can give you the amount of exercise you require.

Professor Sharma had explained to me that even small amounts of exercise were good for you. But was it possible, I wondered, to have too much exercise? I'd had my own health issues when training for the London Marathon – the wandering pacemaker that I'd been told would be fine, but which had led me to lay off the very intense interval training I'd been doing – and I wondered how common these issues were. I had certainly read scare stories in the papers about people suffering ill effects, or even dying, from running the marathon. I was asking the right person: Professor Sharma, on top of everything else, is the medical director for the London Marathon. He explained that the next marathon would see the participation of their millionth runner. Since the inaugural marathon in 1981, and out of those million runners, there had only ever been 13 deaths, which is an absolutely minuscule statistic. So although for a very small number of people, marathon running could be problematic, for most it was absolutely fine.

People are sometimes cautious about a method of exercise known as high-intensity interval training (HIIT) – exercise performed in very brief, very intense sessions. However, I learned that it is only harmful for people with a recognised heart condition. About 1 in 300 young people in the UK has such a condition, and they are usually advised not to engage in HIIT. If people start getting chest pains or feeling faint during HIIT, they should get their heart assessed by an expert before continuing. Otherwise, it's a good way to exercise: there is convincing evidence that 20 minutes of high-intensity exercise three times a week is as good as doing 30 minutes of regular exercise five days a week. This is good news when it comes to the 'time' barrier I've come across before.

The takeaway message was this: too much of anything is bad for you. Too much water is bad for you; too many vitamins can wreak havoc with your body. It's the same with exercise – there's a certain level that the heart can cope with. But the research of Professor Sharma and others at St George's Hospital shows that you need to be exercising quite intensely for 35 years of your life before you even start to show signs of harming your heart. Otherwise, the effects of exercise are overwhelmingly positive.

My conversation with Professor Sharma left me in no doubt about the positive health effects of regular physical activity. And yet it still seemed clear to me that, even when people understand these benefits, they very often still remain physically inactive. I had a theory that a lot of this was to do with confidence.

In the course of my job as a musician in the band, I come into contact with a lot of girls and young women in their teens and twenties. I am always amazed how insecurity and lack of confidence is rife among this predominantly female fan base. This has become more obvious in recent years with the advent of smartphones, social media and selfies. Very often, when fans ask for a selfie with me, they make a point of only putting one side of their own face into the picture. Alternatively, they cover the bottom half of their face with their hands. When I ask them why they do this, the replies always take the same form. 'I'm ugly, so I hide my face.' 'I hate my smile, so I cover it.' The 'half-face selfie' has become a bit of a joke between me and some fans.

Except, of course, it's not really a joke at all.

I do my best to encourage these fans to have more self-esteem.

I ROUTINELY TELL THEM SOMETHING I GENUINELY BELIEVE TO BE TRUE: THAT CONFIDENCE IS ATTRACTIVE, AND IT DOESN'T PAY TO BE OBSESSED WITH YOUR APPEARANCE. THAT I MUCH PREFER A SMILE TO A POUT!

But it's difficult, especially in this era of social media. Anybody with a smartphone is a click away from pictures of the type of person who will create the perfect photo of themselves, with the perfect lighting, the perfect make-up and, of course, the perfect Photoshopping. They present highly curated versions of themselves that are of course unachievable in everyday life. If you lack confidence in the way you look, that must be a very demoralising and demotivating world in which to live.

As a new father, that's not the kind of world I want my daughter to grow up in. I found myself wondering if there was a link between this phenomenon and an alarming statistic that I'd become aware of, namely that there is a massive drop-off in physical activity among girls when they hit the age of 13 or 14. I decided to meet with someone who is not only an expert in the fields of fitness and general health, but who has also taken on the challenge of delivering this message to that hard-to-convince demographic. That person is Dr Zoe Williams, and I found our conversation truly motivating.

You might recognise Dr Zoe. As a GP she's a regular on the *This Morning* sofa and she's a member of the BBC's *Trust Me, I'm a Doctor* team. Unlike most GPs, however, she has an unusual fitness pedigree, having been not only a Premiership rugby player, but also one of the Gladiators – namely Amazon – on the TV show of the same name. Zoe's as cool a GP as you'll ever meet and her story of how she first got into exercise, and of the great help it has been to her throughout her life, is one that I think many people would find inspiring.

Zoe explained to me how she had quite severe asthma as a child – severe enough to warrant being hospitalised on several occasions, and for her life to have been endangered by the condition. Her mum decided that Zoe needed to get some regular exercise in order to help with her lung capacity. Zoe, however, was a super-shy child. She would scream if anybody she didn't know came near her, and her mum had grown quite worried about how withdrawn she could be. In order to find an activity that would help her health and her shyness, Zoe's mum got her into disco dancing.

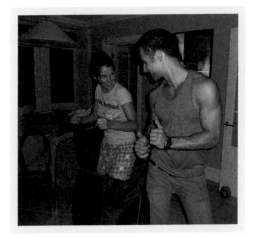

I was fascinated to hear this – not only because I love to dance, but also because part of the philosophy I was developing is that physical activity shouldn't be limited to what people think of as traditional 'sports'. Zoe found that she loved dancing, but it was not without its hurdles. She recalled the anxiety of doing her first solo dance competition – I could certainly relate to that! She lost her rhythm and had to run off the stage, and it took some time for her to pluck up the courage to do it again. But she did and she improved. And although it became too expensive for her to continue once she reached a certain level, she found she had the bug for physical activity. She was constantly encouraged to get out there and be active and, having been introduced to exercise through dance, found herself enjoying all the more traditional sports such as athletics, hockey and netball.

She would still get nervous, but through exercise came confidence – not only in sport, but in other parts of her life. Zoe thrived academically and made it to university where, as well as studying medicine, she competed in rugby to a high level. I was particularly struck by what she had to say about not only the health benefits but also the social benefits of being involved in such an intense team sport. She explained that a lot of the friendships she valued the most to this day were with girls she'd played rugby with. She found that her rugby teams were made up of girls of all different shapes and sizes, or people from private boarding schools playing alongside those from working-class backgrounds. When they all came together to play rugby, none of that stuff mattered. They were a team. The boost to a person's confidence, to their general sense of well-being, that comes from being part of such a unit is surely immeasurable, quite aside from the other physical health benefits.

Zoe was asked to become a Gladiator having applied to be a contestant on the show. She is quite clear, however, that without the confidence she gained from physical activity, she would never even have applied for that first audition. Now she is a regular on TV, a far cry from that shy little girl who would burst into tears if a stranger spoke to her, and an incredible example of how being active can have wide-ranging benefits in all parts of your life. Hearing this from someone else who had experienced these benefits was giving me confidence in my belief in the power of exercise.

Now one of Zoe's passions is going into schools and talking to 14- and 15-year-old girls about all the ways in which bringing exercise into their lives can help them, just like it has helped her. The reasons this age group tend to shy away from exercise are many and complex. They include issues of self-esteem and body confidence at a time when their bodies are changing. They don't like to be seen sweating. They worry about the competitive nature of 'sport' and of feeling self-conscious in front of boys. But when Zoe explains to them that physical activity need not include competitive sport, and that a girls-only Zumba class bestows all the benefits of a game of netball, that physical activity is something everyone can do at their own level and that really nobody can fail at, the response is fantastic. Girls who previously showed little or no interest in physical activity have started to engage with it and girls who were already very active sportswomen have started to appreciate that they can, like Zoe, incorporate it into a successful career. Where teachers and healthcare professionals have struggled to get the message across, Amazon from *Gladiators* is surely making her mark!

It was so inspiring listening to Zoe talk about the power physical activity has to improve the lives of these young girls, but the more we spoke, the more I realised that the importance of her message has far more wide-reaching consequences. I suppose we're all aware that there is a problem with childhood obesity and of course it's important that young people should understand the benefits of exercise. But it's becoming increasingly apparent that, by the time a child is born, it could already be too late. We should be encouraging mums-to-be to get into exercise before they even conceive. This is not only because a child's general health is likely to be influenced by his or her environment, and if the child's parents are not making healthy lifestyle choices, the child has little chance of doing so either. It turns out that a lack of physical activity and poor nutrition can actually change the way genes will work in the unborn child. I was astonished to hear this – I had thought that our genes were fixed, no matter what. Recent research, however, suggests that our genes undergo a process called 'methylation'. This is when methyl groups get added to the end of the baby's genes as a result of the mother's lack of physical activity and poor diet. This in turn affects their offspring – not necessarily when they're children, but as they reach their twenties when they are more likely to suffer from diabetes and obesity.

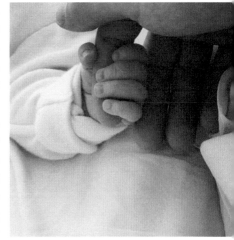

As a new parent, I felt certain that anyone and everyone thinking of starting a family would want to know that your level of physical activity pre-conception could have an impact on your child's future health and well-being. It made me even more determined to get this important message out there in any way I could.

Zoe's interest is not only in educating teenage girls. As part of her campaign to get people active, she also lectures to other GPs and healthcare professionals about physical activity. She finds that a surprising number of them are unaware of the extent of the benefits it can bestow, particularly for people suffering from depression and anxiety, because it has historically never been part of their training. The information she presents in these lectures was very much in line with what Professor Sharma had told me.

WHAT IF THERE WAS A SINGLE PILL THAT COULD REDUCE THE RATES OF PREMATURE DEATH, HEART DISEASE, TYPE 2 DIABETES, COLON CANCER, BREAST CANCER AND ALZHEIMER'S BY MORE THAN 20 PER CENT? WHAT IF THAT PILL HAD NO NEGATIVE SIDE EFFECTS AND A WHOLE HOST OF BENEFICIAL SIDE EFFECTS? WHAT IF IT WAS FREE AND AVAILABLE TO EVERYBODY? WOULD THEY PRESCRIBE IT?

No prizes for guessing what their reply was. And that 'miracle pill', of course, is exercise.

I was interested to understand from a scientific point of view why exercise is so good for you. I had heard about 'endorphins' of course, and had done a little research of my own into what they are. Here's the low-down, in layman's terms. Endorphins are a class of molecules (there are four different types) that our body produces to block pain. They're not only released when we get hurt, but also when we laugh, when we have sex or – importantly – when we exercise. They affect us in the same way as certain opiates such as morphine or codeine, but without the problem of addiction. The part of our brain that handles our emotions is called the limbic system. The limbic system is full of 'opioid receptors'. When our body produces endorphins and they hit these receptors, we experience feelings of pleasure and satisfaction. They stop the transmission of pain signals and stimulate a feeling of euphoria. So, when people talk about vigorous exercise giving them an endorphin hit, there really is something going on in the brain to make them feel better.

There are other hormones and chemicals that the body produces, such as cortisol, dopamine and serotonin. They all affect our mood in different, very complex ways. As with the study of endorphins, the study of these other chemicals is ongoing, but the consensus seems to be that exercise can help your body regulate them. I don't pretend to be a scientist or a doctor, but I was fascinated by the way that exercise could stimulate the production of chemicals that could, in turn, have such a profound effect on our mood and on the way we think.

The study of why exercise is so good for your general health is a field of medical research in which there is a lot more to learn, but Dr Zoe explained to me that a particularly interesting area of research was in the study of a condition called 'systemic inflammation'. We all know what inflammation of, for example, the wrist is: when it gets hot, red and swollen. It turns out that our bodies can be in a constant state of chronic, low-level, all-over inflammation. This inflammation is thought to be the root cause of a lot of diseases such as type 2 diabetes, heart disease, some cancers, dementia and Alzheimer's, as well as anxiety and depression. It is caused by inactivity, smoking, lack of sleep and poor nutrition. Conversely, it is relieved by a healthy lifestyle: physical activity, a good diet, lots of water and plenty of sleep. It goes some way to explaining why aspirin and statins, which have anti-inflammatory properties, can be used to lower the risk of certain conditions such as heart attacks and strokes. But by the same token, there have been studies done in people who have had heart attacks that show that regular weekly exercise is as effective as putting stents into their arteries to stop them clogging up again. This sounded to me like a remarkable fact and explained why Zoe, if a patient presents themselves with, for example, raised cholesterol, is as likely to prescribe walking for 20 minutes a day as she is to prescribe statins.

I think this idea of prescribing exercise, which is precisely in line with Professor Sharma's suggestion, is a brilliant one. Exercise is free. It's available to everybody and it doesn't need any special equipment. Imagine the strain it would relieve on our overburdened NHS if everybody were to take the recommended amount of exercise. Imagine the money that would be saved. Imagine the premature deaths that would be avoided. Imagine how much better we would all feel.

And yet … With her doctor's hat on, Zoe gave me some pretty alarming statistics. In England, 20 per cent of men and 25 per cent of women are physically inactive. That means they do less than 30 minutes of moderate intensity physical activity a week. If somebody is essentially sedentary in this way, their chance of suffering from depression increases by 125 per cent.

So what does 'moderate intensity physical activity' mean? It depends on the person. For someone who is generally fit, it would probably be a jog. For somebody who is generally inactive, it's a brisk walk. During the activity, Zoe suggested, you need to feel out of breath enough so that you can 'talk but not sing'. So we're not talking massive physical exertion. That 30-minute goal, however, is an important one, as Zoe went on to explain.

It's recommended that, in order to get the majority of the health benefits of being physically active, people should aim for at least 150 minutes of moderate intensity physical activity (or 75 minutes of high intensity activity) every week. If you walk ten minutes to the train station and ten minutes the other side, five times a week, you've already nailed a majority of that. However, two-thirds of the health benefits derive from the first 30 minutes of activity. So, even if you only manage half an hour a week, the benefits you derive compared to being physically inactive are massive.

But that's still difficult for some people. As a clinician, Zoe finds it very hard to move people from a mindset of 'I can't' to a mindset of 'I can' when it comes to exercise. To do this, she tries to explore with them their barriers to physical activity and their motivations. Often, she finds, the barriers can be turned into motivations. Worried about exercising because you're experiencing pain? Exercise can help treat your illness. Worried that you have nobody to do it with? Do some physical activity and you'll start to make some friends. Worried that doing more exercise will make you eat more or that you'll undo all the good work by bingeing? Actually

THERE IS GOOD EVIDENCE THAT EXERCISE NOT ONLY HELPS YOU MAKE BETTER FOOD CHOICES — SOMETHING I'VE DEFINITELY FOUND TO BE TRUE — IT ALSO HELPS TO REGULATE YOUR APPETITE.

So while you might eat a little more when you've exercised, because you've burned more calories, your appetite is actually more appropriate to your body's needs.

Other barriers are easily broken down. Worried it's too expensive? When was the last time you had to pay to go for a walk in the park? Worried that you don't have time? Physical activity can very easily be built into your day so you really don't have to find much extra time to do it. It's just a question, sometimes, of thinking outside the box. Zoe told me about a study, done some years ago, comparing bus drivers and bus conductors. The bus drivers were sedentary all day, whereas the conductors were on their feet, moving about, going up and down the stairs. The study showed that the conductors were substantially less likely than the drivers to suffer cardiovascular disease. They weren't necessarily more active outside of their jobs, but physical activity was automatically built into their daily routine. It was another reminder to me that physical activity and exercise are not the same thing, and that it does not necessarily have to interfere with your daily life. It's perfectly possible to make very small tweaks to your routine – taking the stairs instead of the lift, walking to the shops instead of using the car, getting off the bus one stop early – and derive all these amazing benefits.

IN FACT, SMALL CHANGES ARE IN SOME WAYS MORE DESIRABLE THAN LARGE ONES BECAUSE THE MOST IMPORTANT THING IS THAT THEY SHOULD BE SUSTAINABLE.

Joining a Zumba class for a year and then going back to your old ways will have very little effect on your health over the course of a lifetime, whereas small changes that become part of your routine for years will have a genuine impact. For me, the takeaway message was something I'd always suspected: that in order to be worthwhile, exercise has to be manageable and it has to be fun. If it's not fun, you'll stop doing it. That means forgetting about any sports that you find boring, difficult or embarrassing, and replacing them with some form of physical activity that you do like, no matter how untraditional it might seem.

AS I SPOKE TO ZOE, I FOUND MYSELF THINKING ABOUT FANS AT A MCFLY SHOW. I PICTURED THEM WALKING TO THE TRAIN STATION AND THEN TO THE VENUE. I PICTURED THEM RUNNING TO THE BARRIER IN FRONT OF THE STAGE. I PICTURED THEM JUMPING UP AND DOWN IN A FRENZY DURING A 100-MINUTE SET.

Little did they know, but they were exercising just as somebody spending that time on a treadmill or a wattbike. They came away feeling good. I'd like to think everyone was happy because they loved the gig, but it's also likely that the exercise they'd just done was a factor in how good they felt – the endorphins will have been flowing!

It doesn't even have to be a sweaty, 100-minute workout. Zoe explained that the smallest unit of moderate intensity exercise that has a proven benefit is ten minutes. If it's vigorous exercise, make that five minutes. What I realised was that it really is possible to slot small stints of physical activity into your life when it's convenient for you. I was determined to build that idea into the fun and accessible fitness plan that was already taking shape in my head.

I felt that everything I was learning chimed perfectly well with my own experiences and with the philosophy that I was beginning to develop. I wanted to persuade people not only that physical activity was crucial for their physical and mental well-being, but also that – as it's quite distinct from sport – they couldn't fail at it. I was more determined than ever to persuade people that you don't have to go to the gym every day, though of course you can follow my workouts at the gym too if you are a fan. That small changes, which are sustainable and which you might be able to maintain for your lifetime, will make a significant difference to your health and well-being. That

IT DOESN'T MATTER WHAT YOU DO OR WHAT PACE YOU DO IT AT. ANY EXERCISE IS BETTER THAN NONE AT ALL.

My conversations with Professor Sharma and Dr Zoe Williams backed up my initial thoughts and experiences and had given me a real insight into the benefits of exercise from the point of view of healthcare professionals. They had made me understand that improvements I had experienced in my own life were fully supported by evidence and science, and that if I could do something to help get that message out there, I could really help people make a positive impact on their lives.

Perhaps the most significant message I had taken away from my research so far was that physical activity didn't have to equate to those activities that we traditionally think of as 'exercise'. This resonated with me because there was a particular form of physical activity that had improved my life for the better in so many ways. That activity was dance, which had entered my life through my participation in *Strictly Come Dancing*. It gave me just the same buzz as more traditional forms of physical activity.

I wanted to find out more about how and why dancing made me feel so great …

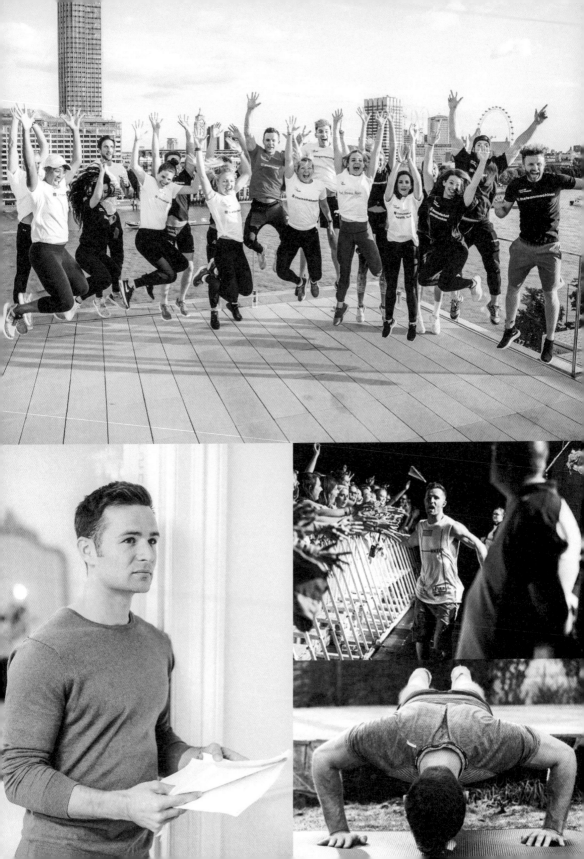

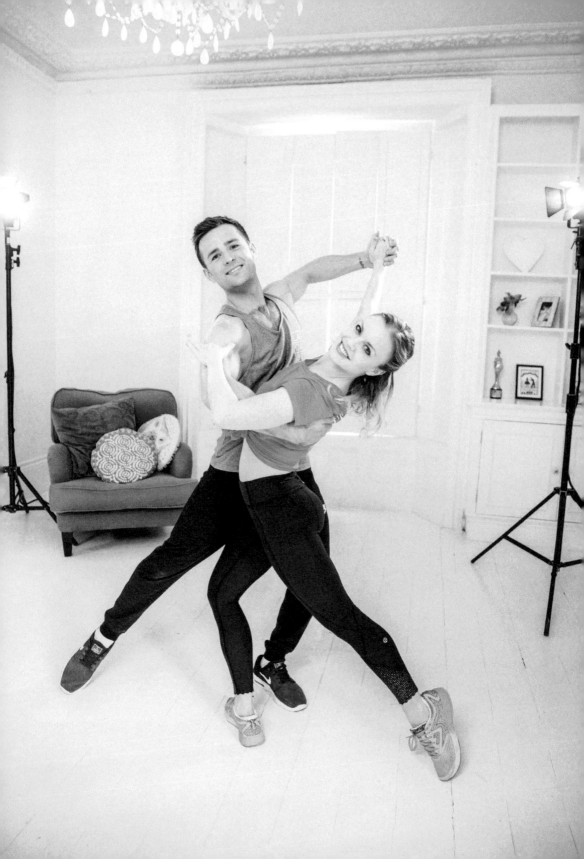

STRICTLY HAPPY

When I was asked to do *Strictly Come Dancing* in 2011, I was very much in two minds. I was still not entirely in control of my anxiety and I was unsure about exposing myself to that level of public attention. It was only after I'd said yes that I experienced my last alcohol-induced panic attack and sheepishly returned to my doctor, feeling a bit stupid, to be reminded that I shouldn't drink as much any more. That was April. *Strictly* started in September. What if my anxiety didn't get better? What if, by putting myself in a position of great anxiety on live TV, I had a panic attack in front of an audience of millions?

The doctor wanted me to recover from that episode naturally, without medication. Thankfully, by the time *Strictly* came around I was fit and well. But I was still, of course, massively nervous. Who wouldn't be? I was no dancer. The first time I got together with my partner Aliona, I was dying inside. Cringing! What would my mates think when they saw me making a fool of myself on TV? What would the public at large think? You know that feeling when you're at a wedding and you're too shy to get up on to the dance floor? Multiply that by a thousand. And the first time I actually had to perform? I get a cold sweat just thinking about it now.

I soon learned, however, that dancing is about letting go and breaking down barriers. Once I'd learned to do that, I found that there was almost nothing I liked to do more. Dancing gave me this incredible buzz, an amazing feel-good factor that was like nothing I'd ever really experienced before. I adored being able to channel music in a whole different way. Most people love music, I think, but learning to move to it and to interpret it takes that love to a whole new level of enjoyment.

WHEN I WAS DANCING, I DIDN'T HAVE THE TIME OR THE INCLINATION TO THINK ABOUT THE ANXIETIES OF LIFE. I WAS IN THE MOMENT, FOCUSING ONLY ON MYSELF AND THE MOVEMENT OF MY BODY.

I was lucky enough to win the show with Aliona and, don't get me wrong, that was an incredible high. But the part of *Strictly* that I loved the most was the rehearsal time. There was no pressure. No audience. Just the dancing. It made me happy. And it wasn't just me who felt that effect. All the other contestants – different ages, different sexes, different fitness levels, different abilities – just seemed to have a big smile on their faces throughout their whole time on the show.

When I returned to do the Christmas Special, having taken some time out from dancing, I couldn't believe how much I enjoyed rediscovering my love of dance. The ballroom dances were always my favourites and it felt like there had been a ballroom-dance-shaped hole in my life. Everything felt good once I was dancing again.

Knowing what I now know about the benefits of physical activity, I guess I shouldn't have been surprised that it had this amazing mood-boosting effect. Dance is physical activity just like any other exercise. But I started to wonder: was there something unique about dancing? Was there something about the movement and the music, about the rhythm and the way you break through your barrier of inhibition, that made dance an especially great way to boost your mood? Was it just me or had anyone seriously looked into this?

Turns out they had. Enter 'Dr Dance'.

Dr Dance's real name is Dr Peter Lovatt. He's a psychologist and Reader in Psychology at the University of Hertfordshire, a great dancer and a serious academic. He is also a living, breathing testament to the power of dance to improve people's lives for the better.

By his own admission, Dr Dance is an accidental academic. He told me that he massively struggled at school. He hated it and seemed to have no aptitude for any of the subjects. He was considered the stupid one. He was unable to read and unable even to be entered for certain exams, let alone pass them. If anyone had suggested that the young Peter Lovatt would one day be a respected academic, they'd have been laughed out of the room.

The one thing he could do, though, was dance. For him, it seemed the most natural thing in the world. It was, in his own words, his reason for breathing. When he danced, he found that his mood was elevated, he thought differently and he felt differently. When he was sitting in the classroom, on the other hand, he felt – his words again – 'thick, stupid and idiotic'. He couldn't read, was very naughty and was suspended and caned a few times – one of those typical bored school kids whose lack of engagement in the classroom manifested itself in his behaviour.

He left school unable to read and with no qualifications – but still with a great love of dance. He went to college to study dance and musical theatre. He then worked in professional theatre as a dancer for several years. By the time he reached his early twenties, however, he still couldn't read.

The turning point came when he was in panto at the Richmond Theatre (as it happens, with my fellow *Strictly* contestant Anita Dobson). He turned up for the two weeks' rehearsal before the show and something suddenly struck him as being not quite right. Looking around the theatre he saw that the actors had their scripts to help them learn their lines. The musicians had their music to read from and a conductor to guide them. The dancers had nothing. They were simply told their moves for a two-hour show and expected to remember them all. There was no chance of writing the moves down, no opportunity to video them as an aide-memoire. They just had to use their memory. Their brains. It occurred to Peter that, if he could learn that amount of content, surely he must be able to learn to read.

And so he did. Taking direct inspiration from his ability to dance, he did what he could never do at school and learned to read. He then took an A level in Psychology. He failed his GCSE English a few times, but eventually managed to get into university to study Psychology and English. He won a scholarship to do his master's and then his doctorate at the University of Cambridge. The rest, as they say, is history: but it was dance that gave him the confidence to take the first step on this amazing journey from being unable to read, to being a serious academic at Cambridge.

Dr Dance's field of academic interest is the psychological effects of dance. When we met he was kind enough to explain some of these to me. I found that what he had to say completely confirmed my belief that dancing is one of the best ways we have to improve our mood, our confidence and our self-esteem.

Dr Dance runs the Dance Psychology Lab, where his team measures a wide range of effects that dance has on the mind. It seems that these effects are profound. He explained to me firstly how dance improves our thinking skills and, in turn, how this can have a great effect on our mood.

There are two types of problem that we routinely encounter in everyday life. The first is the type of problem that has a single answer: 'What is five times seven?' 'What colour is the sky?' The second is the type of problem that has many answers: 'What shall I wear today?' 'What shall I eat?' These second types of problems are called 'divergent thinking tasks'. Typically, we humans are pretty bad at them. We're creatures of habit who easily get stuck into certain ways of thinking that we can't break out of. We might know that we've got a bit of a problem with eating too many chocolate bars, but we find it difficult to apply the divergent thinking we need to break the habit and think of something else to eat.

So what does this have to do with dancing?

It turns out that certain types of dance increase people's ability to use divergent thinking and, in turn, that body movements can be used to break the habits of the mind. Dr Dance has tested this idea in the laboratory, by giving people an ordinary object and asking them to suggest some alternative uses for it – a typical divergent-thinking task. Dr Dance handed me an empty water bottle and asked me to do just that. Apart from thinking that it would be a good toy for Lola, I struggled! Turns out, I'm not alone. In the tests, subjects were generally only able to come up with two or three uses, and they had a tendency for their alternative uses simply to be variations on a single theme. However, if you get the subjects dancing for five minutes – nothing fancy, just improvised movements – they can suddenly find eight or nine original alternative uses for the object in question.

JUST FIVE MINUTES OF DANCING INCREASED THEIR ORIGINALITY AND FLEXIBILITY OF THINKING.

Similarly, it appears to be the case that when people are given numerical tasks that require divergent thinking – like the numbers round in *Countdown* – they tend to do better after a short dance session (maybe offices should encourage dance breaks?). And these effects exist in verbal tests and visual tests too.

So, what groups of people have a problem with divergent thinking?

One group is school children. When they are trying to learn subjects such as Physics or Maths, they often don't think broadly enough. Dr Dance to the rescue. He performed some tests with school children and found that those who engaged in dance activities improved their divergent thinking when they were learning their curriculum.

A second group of people who have trouble with divergent thinking is those who suffer from Parkinson's disease. Dr Dance has found some incredible physical effects that dancing has on this group of people. When they dance, their symptoms are reduced. They find that the day after a dance session, they are able to do simple activities, such as gardening or shopping, that their condition previously made difficult for them. They find it easier to move around the house, they sleep better and consequently they have less pain. But it is not just their physical symptoms that are affected. Dr Dance has also discovered that, when they dance, Parkinson's sufferers experience a significant increase in their divergent thinking skills.

This struck me as very important. Parkinson's sufferers are more prone to depression than non-sufferers. When they dance, they see a marked improvement in their mood, not only just after the dance, but in the long term as well. And it seems clear to me that this might have a consequence not just for Parkinson's sufferers, but for people who need a boost in their mood more generally. It's certainly the case that people with depression experience difficulty with divergent thinking: they might sit on the sofa, knowing what they have to do but finding it difficult to make a decision about how to do it. Changing that pattern of thinking can be hard. But it seems that dancing might be giving us a tool to do just that.

I found myself wondering if, as well as improving people's mood, dancing could also improve their self-esteem. It turns out that this is a more complicated question, although the outcome was not especially surprising to me.

Studies have been done on dancers in vocational training, such as young people in elite ballet schools. The outcome of these studies seems to suggest that people dancing at this level and in that environment have significantly lower self-esteem than pretty much anyone else on the planet. There are two theories about why this might be so. The first is that people who already have low self-esteem tend to be attracted to ballet training because you can almost never be perfect at classical ballet, and this reinforces their poor opinion of themselves. The second is that the ballet sub-culture – whereby you are constantly criticised – is instrumental in destroying a young person's self-esteem.

Further studies have been done where ballet dancers' moods were recorded after they had done a class wearing leotards and tights, and then after doing a class wearing regular baggy tracksuits. They felt significantly better about themselves when they were wearing tracksuits. A similar study looked into the effect of the use of mirrors as part of dance training. When mirrors were present, the dancers felt worse than when they danced without mirrors.

Yet another study looked at professional ballroom and Latin dancers during a competition, when they might have to perform ten different dances throughout the day. Their levels of the stress hormone cortisol were tested throughout the day, and an increase in cortisol was recorded as the competition progressed. The researchers argued that the fear of being negatively judged changed the dancers' social evaluation, increasing their stress levels.

So does all this mean that dancing isn't good for your self-esteem? Not a bit of it. It simply means that the type of dancing you do is important. There are plenty of studies that show that recreational rather than vocational and professional dancing leads to a definite improvement in self-esteem. One such study looked at teenage girls in a school, who rotated between six weeks of swimming and six weeks of dancing. The study found that there was a significant increase in self-esteem after the girls danced. I was reminded of Zoe Williams's message to teenage girls that a girls-only Zumba® class bestows all the same health benefits as a game of netball. Maybe, when you take self-esteem into account, it bestows even more.

Dr Dance explained that different types of dance affect our mood in different ways. Our emotional state influences the way we move. This makes sense – I'm sure that if you were to watch your best friend walking down the street, you could tell a lot about their state of mind by the way they were walking; whether their head was down or their shoulders hunched up. It turns out that this works the other way round – that the way we move affects our emotional state. If we move in a way that we naturally associate with having a low mood, it's likely to induce that kind of mood.

All this is good news for the 'dad dancers' out there! If you're one of those guys (or girls …) who are happy to dance like no-one's watching, arms in the air and body moving all over the place, you're doing just the right thing to make yourself feel great.

This research also chimed perfectly with my own experience on *Strictly*. During my time on the show, the day I enjoyed dancing the most was invariably a Wednesday. Sundays, Mondays and Tuesdays were stressful because I'd be learning a new dance, worrying that it wasn't right and panicking that I wasn't good enough. By Thursday we were leading into the dress rehearsal on the Friday – stressful enough in itself – and the live show on the Saturday. But Wednesdays were perfect. I'd have learned the dance and would just be running it over and over. There was no stress and that meant I enjoyed the dancing all the more.

I experienced something similar during the final. The build-up to that show was immense. It took place at the Blackpool Tower Ballroom, the home of ballroom dancing. Crowds were spilling in to the venue. It was being broadcast live in 3D for the first time. I'd spent the whole week learning three new dances and remembering an old one. I'd messed up my quickstep in the dress rehearsal and, to top it all off, the finalists were supposed to kick off the show entering on chariots dressed as gladiators! So, no pressure …

As I waited backstage for the show to start, my anxiety kicked in. I couldn't focus. I couldn't compose myself. I couldn't really function. Everyone else was furiously preparing themselves to go on stage, but with 20 minutes to go I couldn't even get it together to have a shave. I felt like I couldn't cope. I felt like I was going to buckle under the pressure.

Ten minutes to go. I was sitting in my dressing room, terrified. My mind was scrambled.

I couldn't think my way through the dances I had to perform live on TV any moment. I heard Izzy calling my name – she was worried about me – and I almost collapsed into tears. I felt like breaking down and saying I couldn't do it.

But of course, I had to. I thought of what I knew my mum would say, 'come on, you can do it. Get up, get out there and give it your best, that's all you can ask of yourself.' It was the kind of tough love she gave me when I was nervous about a cricket match when I was younger.

The show started. My first dance was the quickstep. The opening ten seconds of the dance were very complicated. But as I got through them, I saw my mum smiling in the audience. A wave of relaxation came over me.

SOMEHOW, I MANAGED TO SHED ALL THE ANXIETY THAT HAD BEEN BUILDING UP INSIDE. AS SOON AS THAT HAPPENED, I STARTED DANCING THE BEST I EVER HAD.

Over the next three dances I was able to enjoy every moment and really perform. Why? Because I'd managed to let go.

So this is why Dr Dance's theory that we need to shed our anxieties about dancing in order for it to be beneficial to us really rang true. That evening was one of the best of my life – but only once I'd allowed myself to relax, to enjoy myself and to stop worrying about being judged and it going wrong.

There's a big problem with encouraging people to dance and it is this: so many people believe they simply can't do it. They think they're not musical enough. That they don't know where the beat is. Dr Dance told me about some fascinating research that suggests this simply isn't true. That we all have a deep, innate understanding of rhythm, hard-wired in us from the moment we're born. This research tells us that even two-day-old babies can feel the beat.

Here's how we know. You take a two-day-old baby and put a special cap on its head that measures its brain activity. You then play the baby some rhythmic music (this can even be done while the baby is asleep). When the baby is used to hearing the rhythm, you then take a beat out every now and then. Whenever there is a missing beat, the brain responds in a particular way. The baby is expecting the beat, it doesn't happen and the consequence is a 'Where's the beat?' response in the brain.

Bottom line: everyone knows where the beat is. Even babies.

This didn't really come as a surprise to me. From the moment Lola was able to stand up while holding on to something, she would start swaying whenever we played music to her. She particularly loved to bop up and down to 'The Bare Necessities'. We hadn't taught her to do it – it was instinctive. The first time she laughed was when Daddy sang her a Beatles song (thanks Lola!). Babies have no inhibitions and don't hide what they're feeling, and it's obvious to me from the way she smiles and dances to music that she's having a lovely time listening to it.

WE'VE SHARED MANY HAPPY MOMENTS AS A FAMILY THAT HAVE INVOLVED THE THREE OF US DANCING AROUND TOGETHER ON THE KITCHEN TILES. AND WHAT CAN I TELL YOU – SHE LOVES MCFLY!

When Dr Dance and I met, he had recently undertaken a big survey asking mostly men why they don't dance. The most common reason was that they felt self-conscious: they feared being watched, judged and getting it wrong. But they would also frequently say things like: 'I just can't feel the beat' or 'I'm not coordinated enough.' However, as soon as Dr Dance got them into the dance lab and helped them get rid of all that anxiety and tension, it turned out that they could feel the beat and they could get coordinated. It made me suspect that this natural sense of beat perception that has been observed in two-day-old babies doesn't disappear entirely. It just gets buried under a fear of ridicule and failure. If you dig deep enough, I reckon it's not so hard to find.

It's worth mentioning one more study that Dr Dance told me about, the outcome of which is, if anything, even more remarkable. It points to the incredible conclusion that babies' sense of beat perception seems to improve their sociability and the way they interact with the world. In this study, babies of about six months old were bounced on their mums' knees while their mums were either listening to music with headphones on and bouncing them on the beat, or not listening to music and bouncing them randomly. The babies were then taken into another room where a researcher was involved in a task that involved hanging items on a washing line with pegs. The researcher would drop a peg and it was found that the babies who were bounced on the beat were much more likely to pick up the peg and hand it to the researcher than the babies who weren't bounced on the beat. (I had witnessed the same behaviour in Lola. I like to think that when I dance with her, I dance on the beat – and she's forever picking pegs out of the basket and passing them to Granny when she is putting the washing out!) The researchers suggested that moving rhythmically on the beat promotes social bonding and cohesion. Rhythm, and the way we move our bodies, changes how we interact with each other from a very early age.

This struck me as an astonishing finding. But maybe I shouldn't have been astonished. I'd experienced first-hand the power of dance to make me feel less anxious, more energised and better about myself. I'd seen it happen in other people, too. My conversation with Dr Dance was bringing me round to the conclusion that this observation was backed up by science. The right kind of dancing, in the right kind of environment, makes you think better, behave better and – crucially – feel better.

From my discussion with Dr Dance, one thing was becoming clear: there was no way I wanted to encourage people to dance in a situation where they felt they were being judged or where they felt there was any onus on them to look amazing. That would be demotivating, demoralising and simply not what dancing should be about. It should be fun, liberating and energetic. There should be no competitive element – not even a feeling that you're competing against yourself. It should sometimes be challenging enough to be interesting, but essentially impossible to get wrong, because who really cares if you put your foot in the wrong place while busting some moves in the bedroom?

And what about those people who feel that they can't dance? Well, I hoped to persuade them that really, dancing and beat perception are innate in all of us from day one. All we have to do is unlock our inner child!

In fact, there's a great deal we can learn from children when it comes to the benefits of physical activity. I've already explained how, as a child, I was never happier than when I was charging around. Conversely, when I didn't have the opportunity to charge around, my concentration and general behaviour suffered. Perhaps this was why, when I was sitting at home recently watching the *Pride of Britain Awards* ceremony on TV, a particular section really jumped out at me.

There are so many inspirational segments on that show, but among all the stories of bravery, one really made me sit up and listen. An award was given to Elaine Wyllie, the head teacher of a primary school in Scotland called St Ninian's. The reason for the award was that she had introduced an activity into the curriculum that had become known as the 'Daily Mile'.

It's simple but brilliant. At any time during the day, a class teacher can call the Daily Mile. The kids drop whatever they're doing, leave the classroom and run – or walk – a mile. It costs nothing, it's integrated into the school day, it requires no equipment and the beneficial effects seem to be profound. I was completely enthralled by this. I knew I had to find out more.

So a few days later I called the school. A friendly Scottish lady answered. I asked if I could speak to the head teacher.

'Who's speaking?'

'Harry Judd.'

Silence. Bit awkward. I tried dropping the McFly bomb. More silence. Then I played the *Strictly* card. The penny dropped. Phew.

I explained that I had been inspired by what I'd seen about the Daily Mile and wondered if I might come up to Scotland to learn a little more about what they were doing, and the effect it was having on the kids. So off I flew to Scotland to chat to the teachers and the children. What I saw there seemed to confirm everything else I'd learned and experienced about the benefits of a little regular physical activity.

The teachers tended to call the Daily Mile either when the children were becoming a little lethargic or when they were getting overexcited and not really concentrating. Getting outside for some fresh air and a run or walk had a positive effect on both these issues. If they were lethargic, it energised them. If they were overexcited and lacking focus, it calmed them down and helped them concentrate. Only ice or very heavy rain prevents them from taking the 15 minutes required to do the mile.

Most importantly – as I witnessed first-hand by running the Daily Mile with the kids – the children enjoy it and accept it as part of their daily routine. It helps that they don't need to faff around with getting changed or showering. And this simple intervention – easy to implement and completely free – was ensuring that these young people were not only experiencing the short-term benefits of physical activity, they now had the chance of improved health outcomes for the rest of their lives. The reported benefits of academic success, improved confidence and better discipline aren't bad side effects either!

And if these principles worked for kids, I saw no reason why they shouldn't work for adults too. 'Sitting disease' is a real thing – a genuine concern for office workers or other people who spend large quantities of their day sitting down.

SITTING DISEASE IS ASSOCIATED WITH A 112 PER CENT HIGHER RISK OF DEVELOPING DIABETES AND A 147 PER CENT HIGHER RISK OF CARDIOVASCULAR EVENTS SUCH AS STROKES AND HEART ATTACKS.

Sitting, it seems, really could be the new smoking. But what if office workers, and other sedentary people, could learn something from those kids in Scotland? What if there was a way of building exercise into the working day to mitigate these negative effects? Why should the kids get all the fun?!

Seeing the Daily Mile in action gave me complete confidence that the message I wanted to get out there was the right one: relatively modest amounts of physical activity really can have a massive effect on our health and our mood, no matter what our age or previous level of fitness.

I was nearing the end of my research – I could write so much about all the other people I had met too. Everything I had discovered so far suggested that the positive effects of physical activity that I routinely experience are available to anybody and everybody. But I had one more call to make. I wanted to understand more about how physical activity could help people with genuine mental health issues.

Some people find the phrase 'mental health' a bit scary. I don't think we should, because we all have it. Just as we all have different degrees of physical health, so we all have different degrees of mental health. Our mental health might be great, but, just as we all sometimes have a physical ailment, our mental health can also take the occasional dip. It doesn't necessarily mean we have mental health 'problems'; it might just mean we have a few creases to iron out. I believe that if exercise can help people with more profound issues, it can certainly help those of us who just need a bit of a boost. So in order to find out more about how physical activity helps people whose mental health has taken a dip, I decided I needed to sit down with people from Mind, the mental health charity for England and Wales.

Mind does amazing work providing information and support to people with mental health problems. I figured that if anyone could help me understand the mood-boosting power of physical activity, it would be them. So I met with Jack Holloway and Hayley Jarvis at the Mind offices in East London to find out whether my own experiences were in line with other people's. The answer, it seemed to me, was pretty clear-cut.

It was explained to me that exercise is an incredibly powerful tool in the kitbag of anyone wanting to be mindful of their own well-being. It can build resilience, it can treat and manage mental health problems, and it can act as a powerful preventative measure. At Mind, they hear countless stories of people who take up physical activity, having not been active before, and who, like me, are really seeing the benefits. It seemed to me that these benefits would improve anyone's life, not just those who are ill.

Below are the facts that Mind provided. Physical activity:

★ Reduces anxiety and promotes happier moods – thanks to those feel-good hormones called endorphins.

★ Reduces stress and tension. This is because it helps your body regulate levels of the hormone cortisol, which is linked to stress responses.

★ Promotes clearer thinking. By taking a little bit of time out of your busy day, it helps break the cycle of negative thoughts. When your body gets a little more tired, so does your mind, which makes it calmer and your thoughts clearer.

★ Boosts your sense of self-esteem. You derive a great sense of satisfaction from achieving your physical activity goals, from learning new skills, from seeing your fitness levels improve and – yes – from seeing your body improve too.

★ Reduces your risk of depression. The more active you are, the smaller your tendency towards depression. One study shows that if you go from not exercising at all to exercising three times a week, you reduce your risk of depression by 30 per cent.

★ Increases social inclusion. Or, in other words, it helps you make friends and get together with people. This in turn is good for your mental health and general well-being.

★ Is fun, providing you choose the right activity. The more you do things you like, the happier you're likely to be. While that might sound like an obvious statement, research has shown it to be true.

These last points struck me as particularly important. Since social inclusion is good for our mental health and general well-being, I wanted to encourage people not to necessarily think of exercise as a solitary activity, but as a great way to get together with others. It could be one-to-one, in groups or even virtually – I wondered if social media could have a part to play here. I knew from personal experience how isolating mental health problems can be, how it can feel really hard to connect with the world around you when you're in the throes of an episode of anxiety. I had also personally experienced how exercise can help you break out of these episodes. I was equally fully aware that many people find the idea of 'exercise' a real turn-off. Just because I see the gym as a playground, it doesn't mean everybody does, and I totally understand that some people find gyms completely intimidating. Physical activity has to be fun, otherwise it's simply not going to be sustainable and it's not going to have the same beneficial effect.

Hayley from Mind explained to me that among the most popular activities people with mental health problems are taking part in were the following:

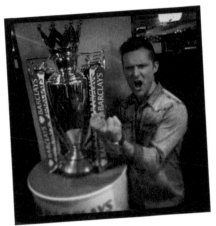

★ Football (an incredibly powerful way of making social connections, whether people wanted to be involved in competitions or simply have a kick-around)

★ Badminton (again, a social, stop-start game where you can chat between rallies)

★ Walking groups (getting outside in the fresh air, taking in the sights, sounds and smells of nature)

★ Boxfit (structured and disciplined, which can help people experiencing mental health problems, and also very stress-relieving)

But Hayley was also at pains to point out that non-traditional physical pursuits had just the same mood-boosting effects as more obvious ones. Think 'ultimate Frisbee', she told me, or boccia, a Paralympic sport a bit like bowls. Anything that gets people moving can go some way to helping with mental health issues. Physical activity of any kind whatsoever is a powerful weapon for those struggling to get their heads in the right place.

For me, the takeaway fact was this: physical activity improves our mood. Anything we can do to introduce it into our lives will make us feel better. Period.

Here, in a nutshell, is what I had learned:

PHYSICAL ACTIVITY CAN KEEP YOU HEALTHY.
PHYSICAL ACTIVITY CAN MAKE YOU LIVE LONGER.
PHYSICAL ACTIVITY CAN GIVE YOU CONFIDENCE.
PHYSICAL ACTIVITY CAN HELP YOU TO CONCENTRATE AND FOCUS.
PHYSICAL ACTIVITY CAN BOOST YOUR MOOD.
PHYSICAL ACTIVITY CAN TREAT AND PREVENT MENTAL HEALTH ISSUES.
GETTING FIT REALLY IS A WAY TO GET HAPPY.

You don't have to do loads of exercise. The recommended amount is 150 minutes a week (or about 20 minutes a day), but two-thirds of the health benefits derive from the first 30 minutes a week. You can break this time down into much smaller units and still reap the rewards.

You do have to enjoy it, because otherwise it won't be sustainable. But fortunately … Anything that gets you moving counts – including dancing!

As a result of all this research I started to put together my Get Fit, Get Happy fitness plan, drawing from all the investigation I'd done and the facts that I'd accumulated. I wanted a plan that was completely simple and enjoyable for people to incorporate into their daily life. I wanted it to be something people could do anywhere – at home, in the park, in the office – and with anyone – a friend, a partner, with their kids or by themselves, of course. I wanted it to be sustainable and fun, not scary and a drag. I wanted it to be accessible enough for people who lack the confidence, the skills or the fitness to take on a hard-core workout, but challenging enough for those who wanted to step things up a little.

Here's what I didn't want: I didn't want it to be an insanely structured, strict or unsustainable fitness plan that makes you feel like you have failed if you miss a workout. I'm not promising an 'eight week' transformation. I don't want to promise to get anybody 'beach-body ready' nor tell you to focus on sculpting this or sculpting that. Because what happens when the eight weeks are over? What happens when the holiday comes to an end?

I wanted my fitness message to be one of balance, sustainability and realistic achievements. Most of all I wanted the focus to be on how much better physical activity makes you feel, rather than how it makes you look. I believe that if you adopt this mindset, you'll soon find the aesthetic benefits show too but without you ever having to worry about them. That's what I want you to remember in the pages that follow. I believe it can be life-changing – it has been for me – because if you approach exercise in a fun way, it will become something that you want to do. I've said it before but you can't fail at exercise and if you do happen to be having a bad few weeks or you are feeling demotivated, you are only ever one workout away from getting back on track.

THIS IS ABOUT HOW YOU FEEL ON THE INSIDE, NOT HOW YOU APPEAR ON THE OUTSIDE. IT'S NOT ABOUT SUCCEEDING OR FAILING. IT'S NOT ABOUT WINNING OR LOSING.

It's about reaping the health and mood benefits, and it's about having fun. Nothing more, nothing less.

I am not cured of my anxiety or my OCD. These are, I think, issues that will be with me for the rest of my life. They are a part of me. I know that if I'm not mindful of my mental well-being, the pressure can build. I'm still prone to anxiety and I know that if I don't take care of myself in other ways, such as exercising, eating properly and getting enough sleep, it can and will get worse.

So, I don't want to pretend that, if you suffer from similar problems that affect your state of mind, exercise is some kind of cure-all, that it will make your problems disappear overnight. It isn't and it won't. Our brains are complex things and the factors that affect them are different for everyone.

But I am certain of this: exercise is the most valuable item in my well-being toolkit. It keeps my anxiety at bay and I know it's always there for me if my problems should start to build. And my research tells me that this can be true for everyone. Getting fit really can help us to stay happy.

With that in mind, I want you to get creative. Maybe the workouts in the next section aren't for you. If so, that's completely fine. You just need to find the physical activity that is for you. I guarantee there's something out there. Perhaps the next few pages will help you find it.

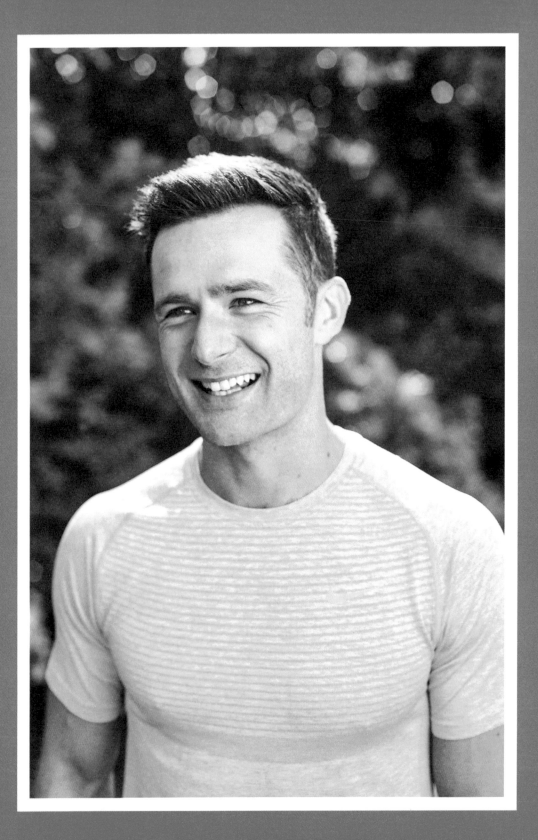

THE GET FIT, GET HAPPY FITNESS PLAN

In the following pages I've combined the results of all my research with my own experiences and instinct to create the *Get Fit, Get Happy* fitness plan to help you get fitter and happier. There's no set schedule, the workouts and dances that follow can be done anywhere, anytime and without any equipment. I'm not setting any unrealistic goals and my main aim is to make exercise fun, sustainable and achievable.

But before we do that, I want you to know that these exercises are a very long way from being your only option. I understand that doing a workout may feel like the last thing you want to do – I know, I've been there – sometimes just getting up and going for a walk feels like a big ask but if you can even just manage that, it's a great start. I want to urge you to think outside the box when it comes to physical activity. I want you to think about stuff that you actually enjoy doing or stuff that you might start to enjoy if the competitive element is taken out. Repeat the mantra: you can't fail at exercise. And if you're worried that you might be too slow to go for a run, remember this: once you're out there,

NO MATTER HOW SLOW YOU ARE, YOU'RE STILL LAPPING EVERYBODY WHO'S SITTING ON THE SOFA!

With that in mind, here are a few ideas to get you moving.

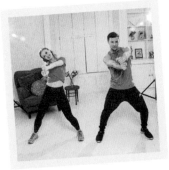

DANCE

On pages 222–251 you'll find some dances I've put together to help you on your way. But there are loads of dance classes all over the country. Trust me, it's amazing exercise. Do a Zumba class and you'll be sweating like the best of them, but an hour of ballroom, or tango, or salsa, or hip hop, or belly dancing, or any kind of dancing is easily as good for your mood and your fitness as an hour in the gym.

If dancing classes aren't your thing, you can get just the same benefit from dancing when you go clubbing (minus the booze). You can even do 'Clubbercise' – an exercise class performed in the dark to dance music – or from jumping up and down at a gig. And you don't even need to step out of the house to do a dance workout. Do it in your bedroom or your kitchen. Stick on your favourite tune and boogie like nobody's watching. I guarantee you'll be getting as good a workout as you've ever had, and you'll finish up with a Cheshire cat grin on your face – and that's what we're aiming for, right?

RUN

Completely free, and everyone knows how to do it: running is the original and best form of physical activity, and it burns more calories than pretty much any other type of regular, mainstream exercise. More importantly, it's hard to beat that post-run high. A run keeps me upbeat and happy for the rest of the day.

You don't have to be Usain Bolt. In fact, you don't want to be Usain Bolt. You just want to work yourself up to a position where you can get a bit out of breath a couple of times a week. Ease yourself in super-slowly by building up your speed and distance gradually. In my experience, going for a run is always a good idea, because no matter where my head is, it always makes me feel better.

If you're lacking in motivation (we've all been there) stick your running shoes on and promise yourself that you'll jog 100 metres before deciding whether or not to turn back. If you decide to leave it there, fine: give yourself a high five for doing more than you thought you would initially. I've got a sneaking suspicion, though, that once you're out there you'll probably want to carry on.

Running with a friend can be awesome, but if you're a beginner it's probably best not to make it that friend who runs marathons for fun. Most running clubs have groups for different levels and they can be a brilliant way to get started and meet new people at the same time.

I'd advise getting a half-decent pair of running shoes if this is going to be your thing.

WALK

Don't underestimate the power of walking. Even if you don't fancy any of the other activities in this book, even if you never go for a run, never do a workout and positively hate dancing – if you start walking a little more than usual, I guarantee you'll start to feel the benefits.

There are so many ways to get a bit of extra walking into your routine. If you walk ten minutes to the train station and ten minutes at the other end, five times a week, that's one hundred minutes of physical activity under your belt. Do you normally stand on the escalator? Walk instead: it really adds up. People who have a dog and walk them daily are undoubtedly getting their weekly exercise fix. Job done (although a dog is for life, not just for 150 minutes a week ...). But you can get creative. Do you have a half-hour meeting at work? Why not make it a walking meeting? Meeting a friend for coffee? Take a couple of turns round the park instead. Walk to the shops. Walk to the pub! Just walk!

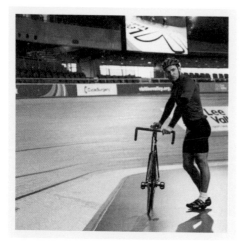

you can hook up with fellow cyclists of all ages and abilities so you can keep motivated and have a laugh with other people.

PLAY VIDEO GAMES

What?

Sure. Why not? I'm not saying that hours and hours in front of a screen is going to do much for your mood, and I'm certainly not saying all video games give you a workout. On the McFly tour bus we always have the latest FIFA game to while away the time and I'm not going to lie: our competitions get heated, but we don't get much exercise. There are plenty of video games that do give you a workout, though. Wii Fit, Wii Tennis, Just Dance, Nike+ Kinect Training … The list is almost endless, and the bottom line is that physical activity is physical activity, whether you're in the park or in front of the Xbox.

CYCLE

You can spend thousands of pounds on bike equipment, but you really don't have to. It doesn't take much to fix the puncture on that old bike gathering dust in your shed or you can pick up second-hand bikes for next to nothing.

And if you think going cycling means you have to be one of those super-fit, super-lean, Lycra-clad dudes you see leading the peloton on TV, think again. A gentle bike ride through the park will boost your mood and your fitness just fine. It's amazing exercise and a brilliant way of getting active with the family or with a bunch of mates.

If you can replace those daily car trips to the shops, or even your commute, with a bike ride, chances are you'll be getting your recommended weekly exercise hit without even thinking about it. And if you want to take things a bit further, there are hundreds of local cycling clubs where

SWIM

Swimming is just about the best exercise you can get. Swimming a few lengths works most of the major muscle groups and gives you an aerobic hit too. Take the kids, splash around with them, have fun. If you want to ramp things up a bit, most public swimming pools have workout classes.

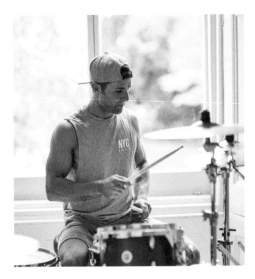

But they're also fantastic ways of getting some physical activity. You can play them with your kids, of course – you'll be laughing along with them before you know it – but there's really nothing to stop you organising a game of good old fashioned British Bulldog in the park with your adult mates. In fact, there are lots of groups of adults up and down the country who do just that. It's a great way to get fit while making new friends and keeping up with old ones.

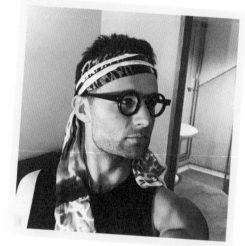

PLAY THE DRUMS

Works for me! An hour knocking the hell out of the kit is as good a form of exercise as I know: it's fun and it keeps your brain engaged as well as your body. Of course, it doesn't have to be the drums: there's good evidence to suggest that playing the violin for an hour burns the same number of calories as walking for an hour at a moderate pace (Izzy reckons it's because of the brain power involved!). So if there's an instrument you used to play as a kid, pick it up again.

PLAY LIKE A KID

There's a reason all those childhood games – I'm talking Tag, British Bulldog, Capture the Flag, Grandmother's Footsteps, What's the Time Mr Wolf? – have endured: it's because they're fun.

PLAY CRICKET

(or football, or whatever floats your boat). I've already told you about how I loved cricket as a child. Somehow, when we get older, we imagine that we don't have time for games like that any more. Not always true. My friends and I had talked about putting a cricket team together for years. Finally we did it. We found a league called 'Last Man Stands'. For the cricket buffs among you, it's an even shorter version of 20/20, eight-a-side with five-ball overs. Games start at 6.30 p.m., so it's after work, and you can pick which evenings are best for you all. If you want the competitive element, it's there. If not, it's just a great way of hooking up with your friends, enjoying a bit of camaraderie and adding a bit of exercise into the mix.

It doesn't have to be cricket, of course. Put together a regular game of five-a-side football in the park. Tag rugby. Netball. Rounders. If there's a team game you used to enjoy as a kid, do that. You'll have a blast.

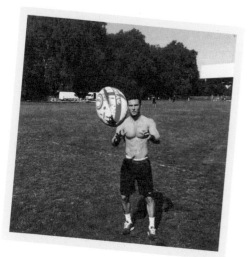

GET A DOG

Obviously a dog's for life, not just for half an hour's exercise, but I've seen first-hand the benefits of having one. My mum and dad live in the country. They've just got

themselves a dog and my mum waxes lyrical about all the benefits it has brought her, because she has to take the dog for a walk every day and it forces her to make the time to do that. Dogs love exercise and that enthusiasm is infectious. All they want to do is go out and chase a ball (a bit like me, really …).

GARDENING

It might sound silly, but gardening is a fantastic way to keep active. My mum and dad do it all the time! All that bending down, digging, raking and pushing your wheelbarrow up and down is brilliant physical activity. I also find it's a great form of meditation, and keeps me in the moment when things are getting on top of me.

SEX

Blushing? Don't. I'm not going to presume to give you any tips, but physical activity is physical activity and it doesn't matter how you get it.

Is it moderate exercise or vigorous exercise? That's down to you. As for how long it lasts…?

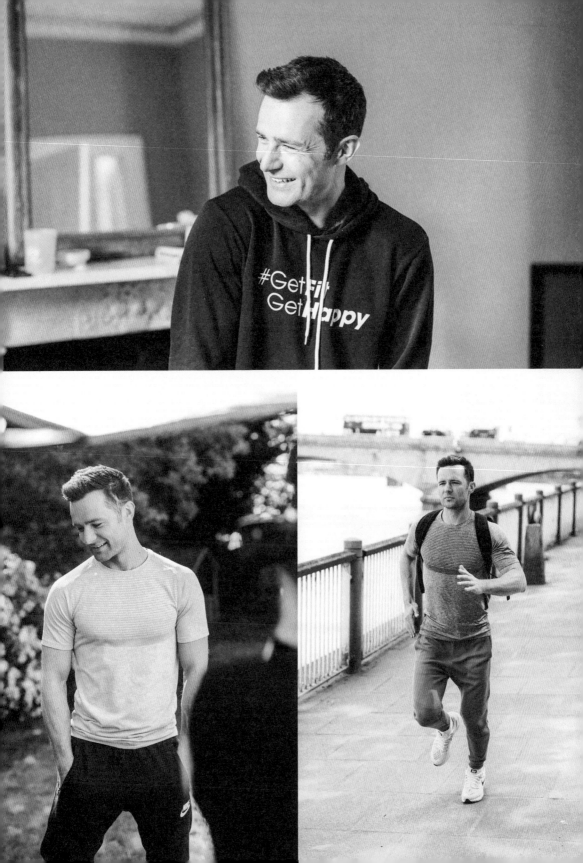

Now I know you are raring to go. S Club is pumping on the stereo, your trainers and headband are on and you're shouting 'Yes Harry! Let's do this!'. But hold up! There are just a couple more things for me to share...

WARMING UP

Before you start any of these workouts, it is important to warm up. Spend 3-5 minutes moving. A good example would be to start by walking on the spot, then marching (bring your arms into it), then jogging and finally running on the spot. You could replicate some of the movements in the exercises in the workout you are about to do to get the right muscles moving. We just want to get that heart rate up, loosen those joints and get your blood flowing to your muscles and you'll be ready to go!

INJURY

If you have an injury or any concerns about your fitness or health please check with a healthcare professional before doing any exercise.

HARRY'S QUICK TIPS

- Always try to engage your core throughout the exercises as it'll help you maintain a good posture and help to prevent injury too. One way to think of engaging your core is to imagine you're bracing yourself for a punch in the stomach. It sounds extreme but it is the best way I can think to describe it!

- When it comes to what tempo to do the exercises at, use your breathing as a guide. For example if you are doing a squat, breathe in on the way down and out on the way up.

- Listen to your body. Don't try and be a hero. If you need to rest, rest because if you power through you'll end up doing more harm than good.

- To keep things simple, I'm suggesting you work and rest for set periods of time. These are just suggestions for different levels of ability but you may find you want to work for different lengths of time or for a number of reps instead.

- Do the best that *you* can do. Don't compare yourself to others. Your sprint might be someone else's jog and that's OK! You might be doing push-ups against the wall while someone else is doing them on the floor one-handed but you're still working just as hard as they are.

- If you are feeling nervous or struggling to find motivation, put some music on (I've heard McFly have some good up-tempo numbers), be positive and most importantly, have some fun.

NOW LET'S GO!

RISE AND SHINE

Here's something for those of you who like a bit of strenuous activity in the bedroom! You can do this first thing in the morning – always a positive way to start the day – and the bedroom's a good place to hide away if it's bedlam in the rest of the house. Next time you feel like a duvet day, try this instead and see how you feel afterwards. All you'll need is a bed and a pillow.

This is a five-minute workout. To increase it to a ten-minute workout try adding the cardio moves on pages 102-103 in between each of the exercises in the workout. If you want to really feel the burn, do two rounds of this for a 20-minute workout.

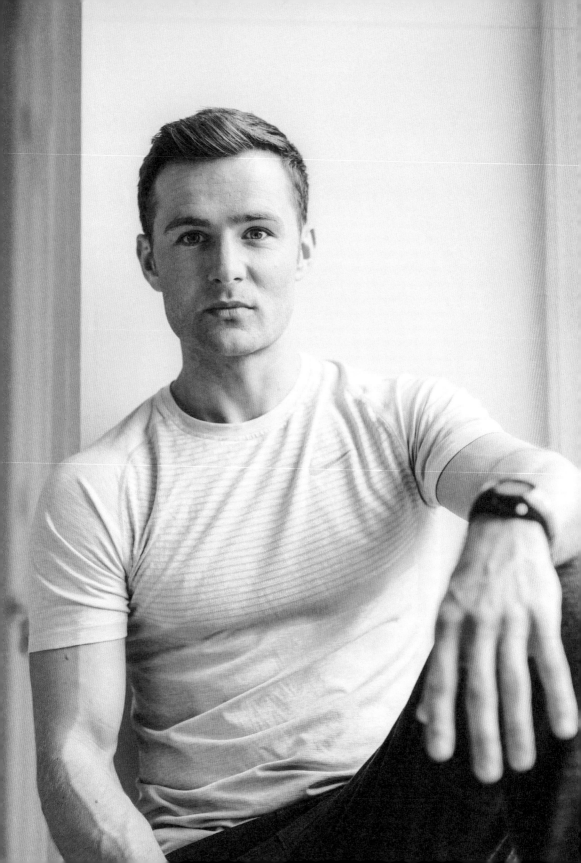

Squat – make sure you keep your heels on the floor and your knees in line with your feet as you tap your bum on the bed.

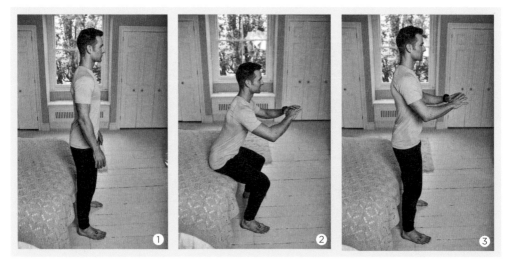

Push-up – place your hands just wider than shoulder-width apart on the bed. Go as deep as you can, even if just a small amount. You'll soon see progression.

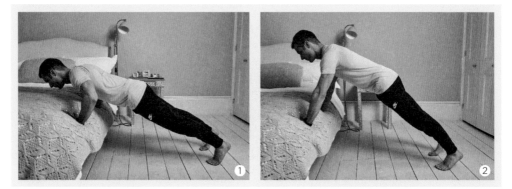

Single leg raise – engage your core and try and keep your legs straight!

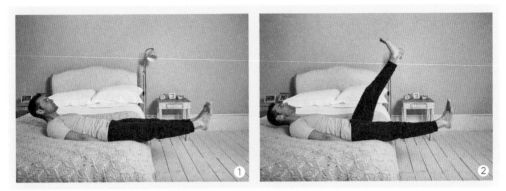

Static lunge – you can hold onto something like a table to help with your balance. 20 seconds on each leg.

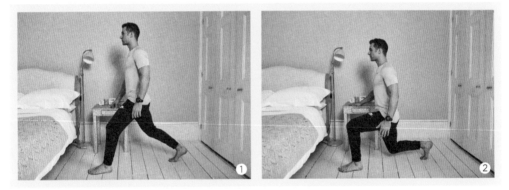

Handstand progression – slightly bend your elbows, stay strong in your arms and upper body and jump up into position 2. Land softly!

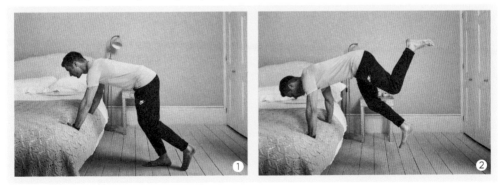

INTERMEDIATE

Squat – still keep your heels flat on the bed and knees in line with your feet but really focus on your balance and stability.

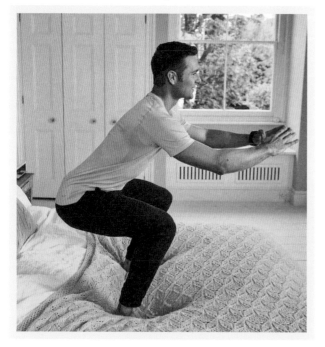

Push-up – you can have your knees on the bed if you can't achieve a full push-up yet.

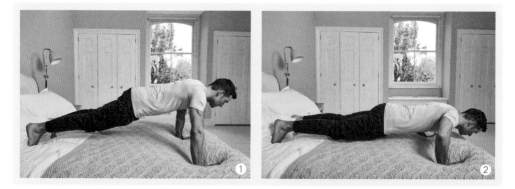

Leg raise – keep your legs together and try to keep your lower back flat on the bed.

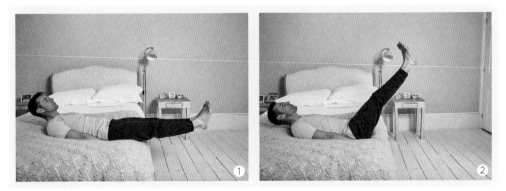

Split squat – focus on balance and don't rush. Keep your weight on the front leg. 25 seconds for each leg.

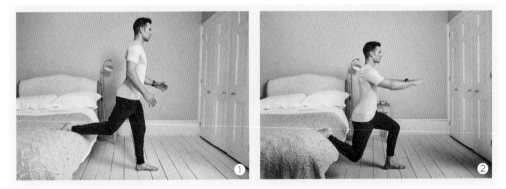

Handstand progression – stay strong in your arms and upper body and jump into position 2. Land softly.

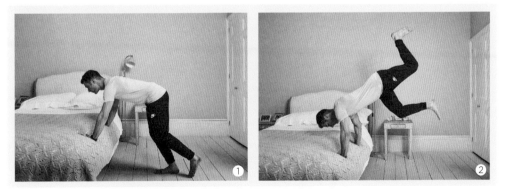

ADVANCED

Perform each exercise for one minute, no rest.

Squat jump – explosive jump with a controlled landing.

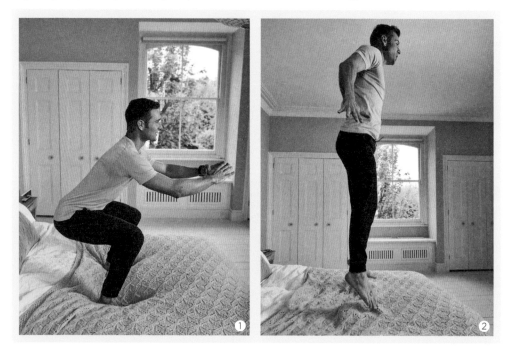

Decline push-up – stay strong my friend! If you don't have a headboard put your feet on the bed and your hands on the floor.

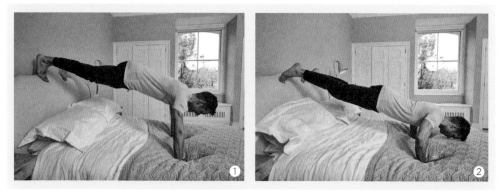

Leg raise into reverse crunch – keep your head slightly off the bed. Feel the burn!

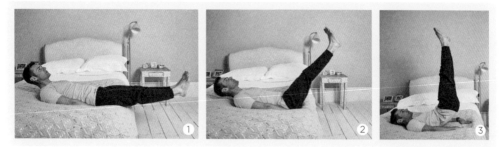

Jumping split squat – 30 seconds on each leg.

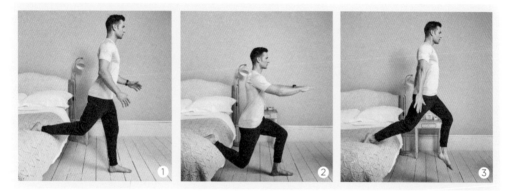

Handstand progression – control required! I've gotten carried away before and gone over – I was certainly thankful for the soft landing on the bed!

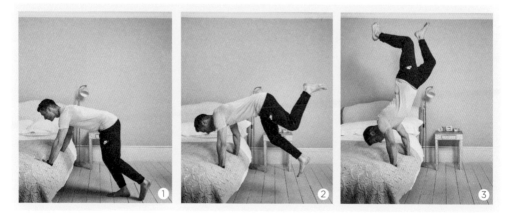

ADDITIONAL CARDIO EXERCISES

Add these five cardio moves in between each strength exercise to increase the length of your workout to ten minutes. For beginners perform each exercise for 40 seconds, rest for 20 seconds. At intermediate level perform each exercise for 50 seconds with 10 seconds rest and for advanced level perform each exercise for one minute with no rest.

Semi-circle mountain climber – To perform a mountain climber get down into a straight-arm plank and drive one knee forwards and then pull it back again. Swap legs. Try moving around in a semi-circle as you go.

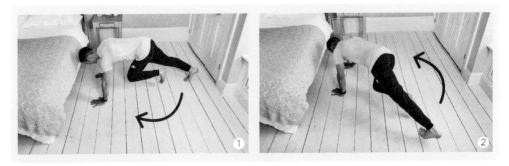

Butt kickers – alternating legs.

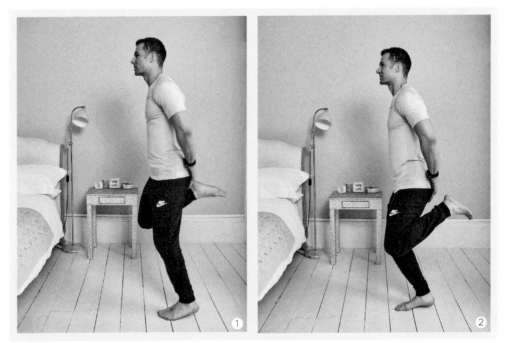

Tuck jump – jump up and keep your knees tucked in.
Focus on achieving a soft landing.

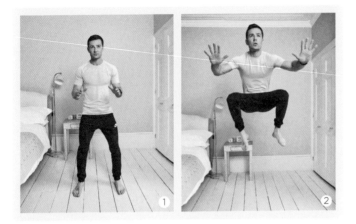

Moving squats – alternate between close squats and wide squats.

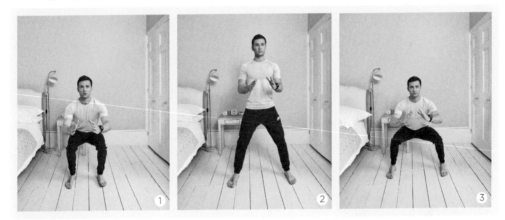

Pillow drills – lay out some pillows or clothes as markers and run sideways
in between them.

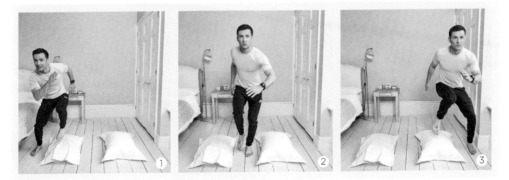

IT TAKES TWO

When I took these photos, Izzy was pregnant, so I borrowed a friend from Strictly — Joanne Clifton. Exercising is a great way for couples to spend a bit of time together. No equipment required — all you need is each other.

Try each exercise for up to a minute factoring in rest time dependent on your ability.

Fireman's lift and squat – advanced movement.

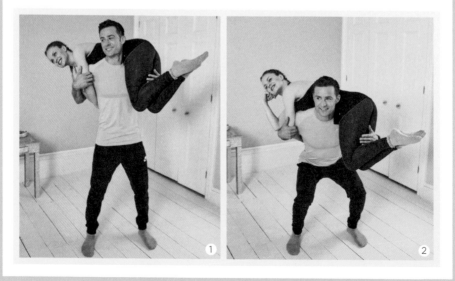

Side plank adduction – try to keep your body straight and that top hip aimed up to the ceiling.

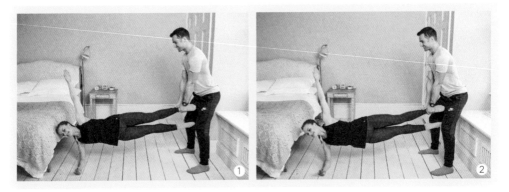

V-sit abduction – the partner with their feet on the outside controls the level of resistance.

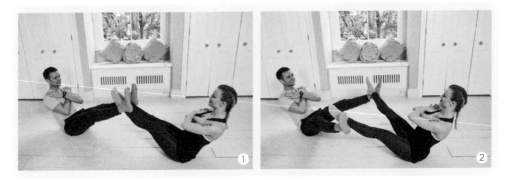

Push-up and deadlift – go down into each respective exercise at the same time.

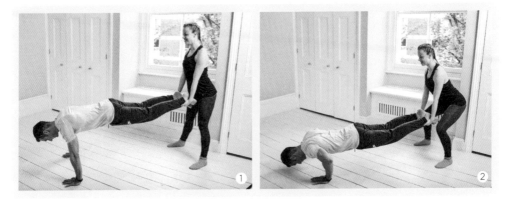

Plank with bridge – the person planking stays static throughout. The person bridging needs to push their hips through and squeeze their bum at the top of the rep.

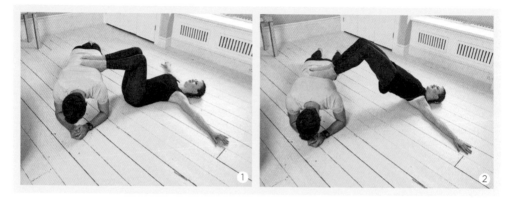

Hamstring curl – this is super challenging. Ease yourself into this one.

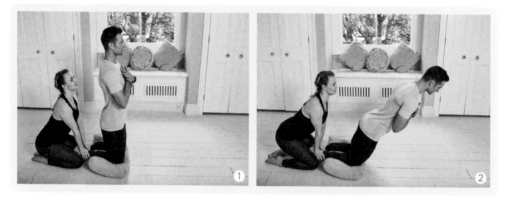

Leg press – the person on the floor controls the exercise. Effective and funny at he same time!

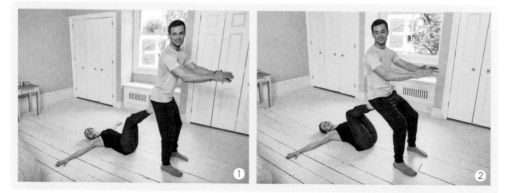

Bridge and dip – the person bridging stays static throughout. If you are dipping you can try straightening your legs to make the dip harder.

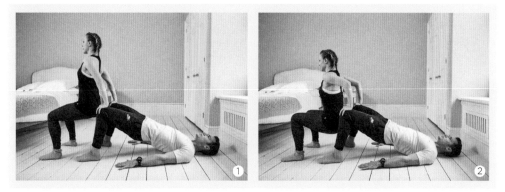

Straight arm plank and hop over

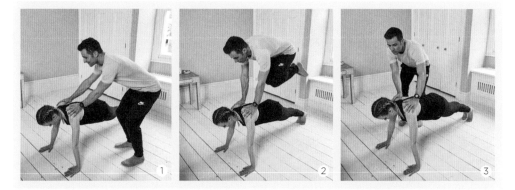

Wall squat and split squat – 30 seconds on each leg for the person squatting or see who can last the longest!

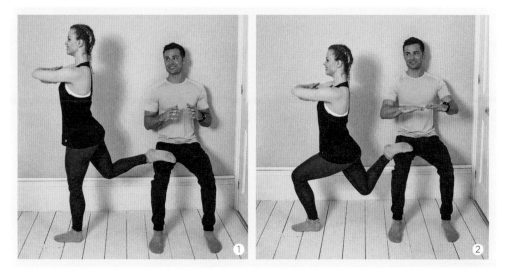

PILLOW TALK

Another couples' workout. For ages I didn't know what the term 'pillow talk' actually meant – Izzy had to explain it to me. Don't tell her, but I think I might prefer this version. There are some fun exercises to try together here. To turn them into a workout try performing each exercise for 30-60 seconds and take a 10-20 second rest between each one, then repeat.

All you need for this is a couple of pillows. Pillow fight optional!

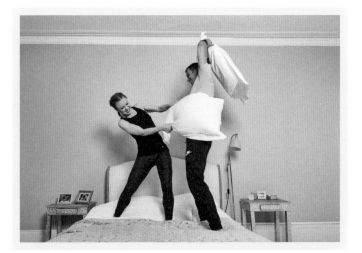

Pillow slam – slam the pillow, pick it back up, Simples.

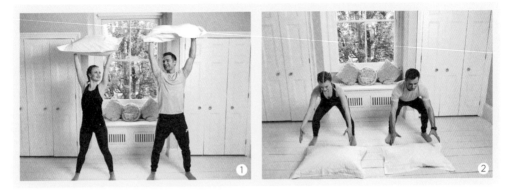

Pillow twist – to make it easier, keep your feet on the floor. Cheesy grins are compulsory.

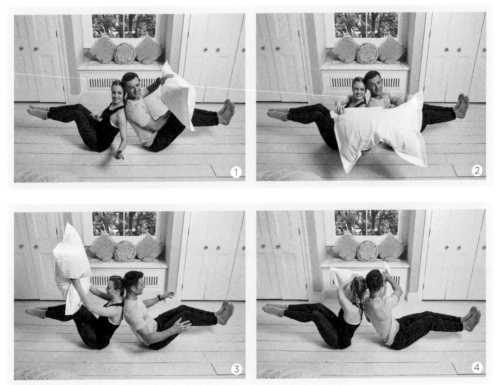

Squat and throw – the power of your throw can be dependent on how annoying your partner has been today.

Burpee and throw – take it in turns.

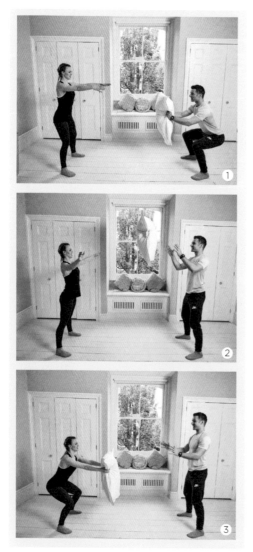

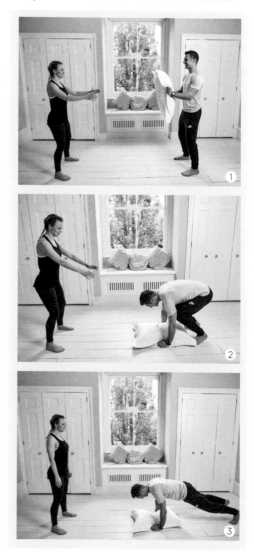

Partner crunches – pass the pillow at the top of each crunch.

Straight arm plank while passing pillows through arms – once pillow gets to the other side, swap arms and pass it back through. Try to keep your hips as still as possible.

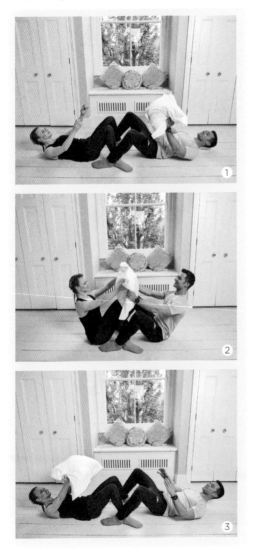

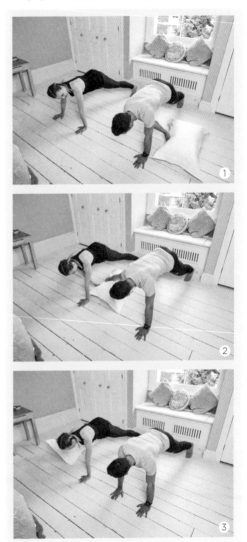

THE STRESSBUSTER

I've talked a lot about how you can feel really great after a workout, I can go into a workout feeling lethargic and come out the other side feeling epic. This workout though is great for those times when you are feeling really stressed or angry and you need an outlet for all that tension. Smash this out and I guarantee you will feel better for it afterwards. Try each exercise for up to a minute factoring in rest time dependent on your ability.

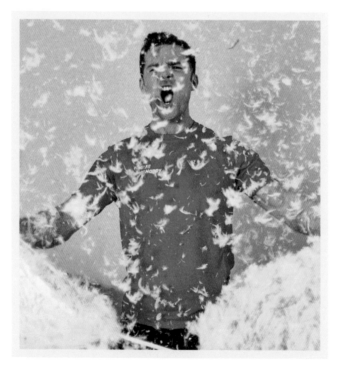

Running on the spot with air punches

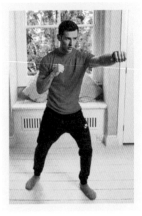

Squats with hooks

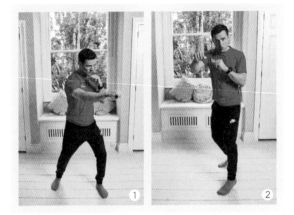

Angry jumps – basically a squat jump but feel free to scream in the air to let out any tension!

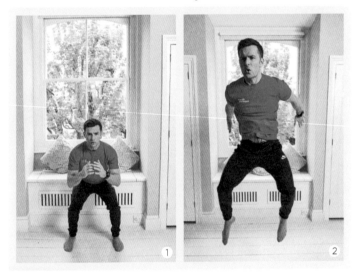

Push up and punch out – push-ups can be done on your knees.

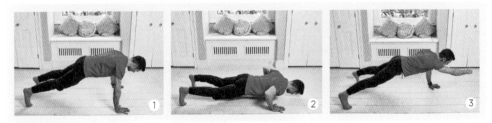

Pillow slam burpees

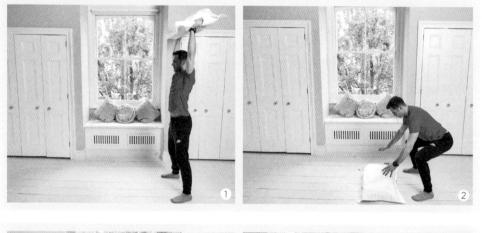

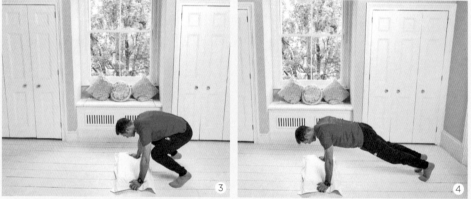

Mountain Climbers

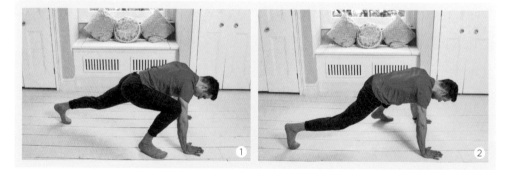

Knee into pillow – teach those feathers who is boss!

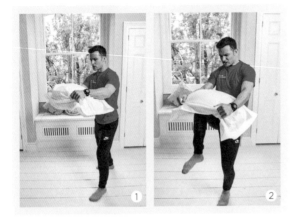

Low to high punches

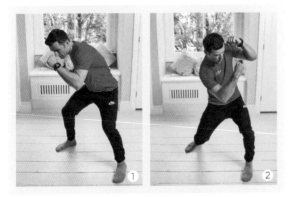

High knees – running on the spot lifting your knees as high as you can (ideally in line with your hips).

Punching a pillow on the bed – feel better?!

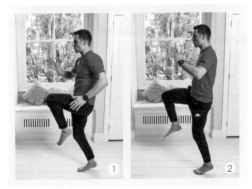

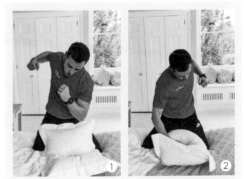

SHOWER TIME

Too busy to exercise? No time? But you have time to take a shower, right? Let's kill two birds with one stone – here are some simple exercises you can do in the shower.

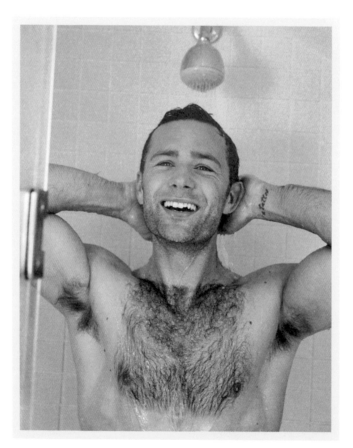

Static squat

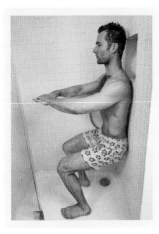

Wall push-up – if you are working towards a full push-up this is a good progression.

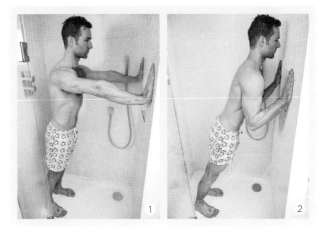

Knees to elbows – bring your right elbow to your left knee slowly, focus on the abdominal crunch. Alternate.

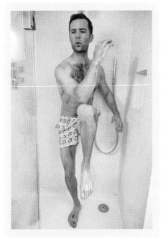

Tricep wall push – move your hands closer in and keep your elbows tucked in close to your sides to focus on your tricep muscles.

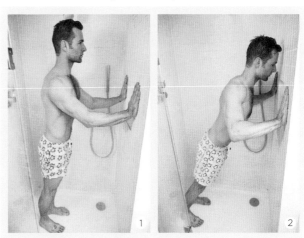

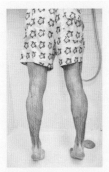

Calf raise – if you suffer from a severe case of chicken legs like me then this is a good exercise for you!

STAIRWAY
TO HEAVEN

If you live in a bungalow, this one's not for you, though there's nothing stopping you finding some steps elsewhere and giving it a go. If you live in a high-rise, then good luck! This is a killer on the legs – no escalators or taking the lift, please.

Work for 30-60 seconds on each exercise with 0-30 seconds rest. N.B. I take no rest #justsaying.

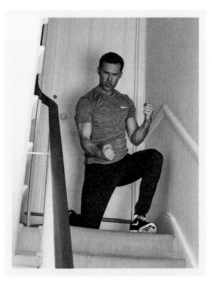

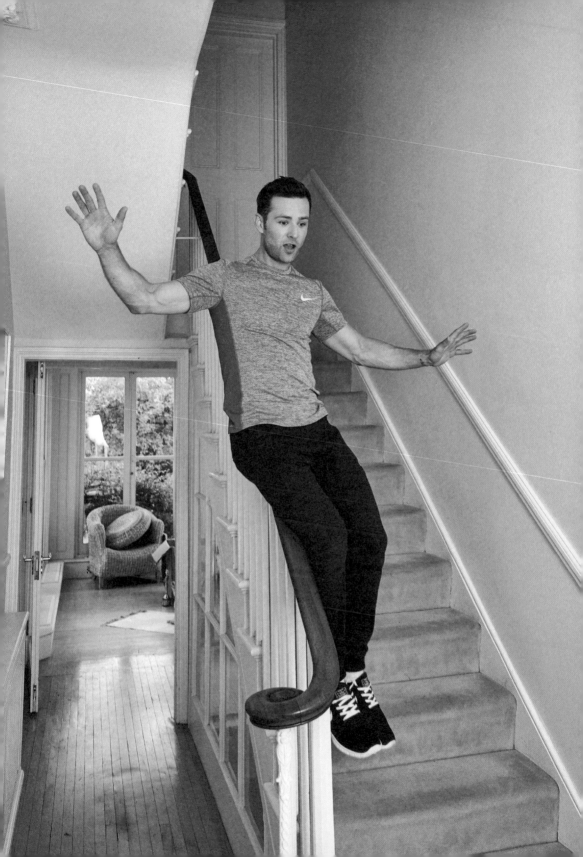

Split lunge (right leg)

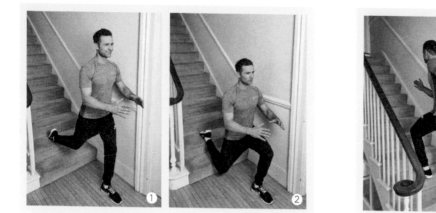

Push-up

BEGINNER – the higher the step, the easier the push up.

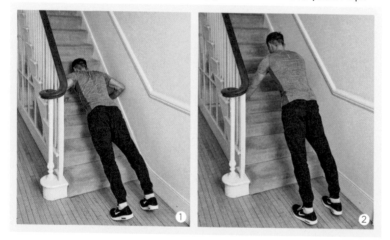

ADVANCED – the higher the step, the harder the push up.

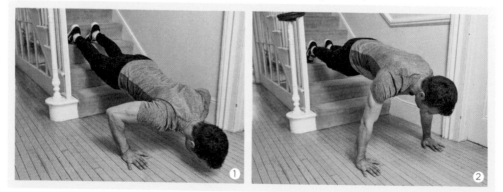

Jump squat – all the way to the top!

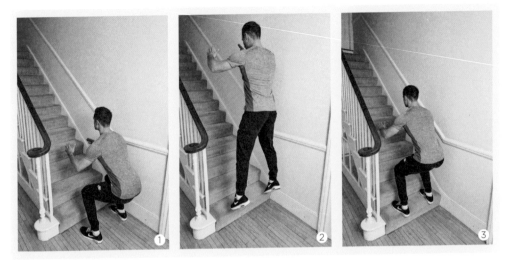

Bridge

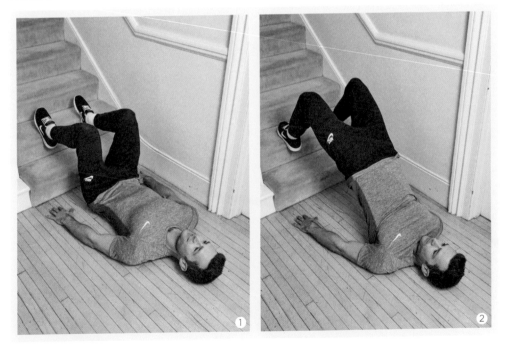

Run up the stairs – two steps at a time.

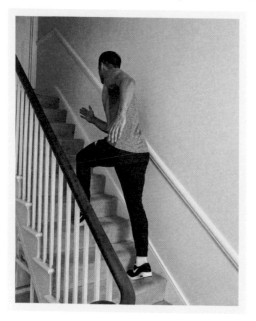

Dip – you can do this with your legs bent or keep them straight to make it harder.

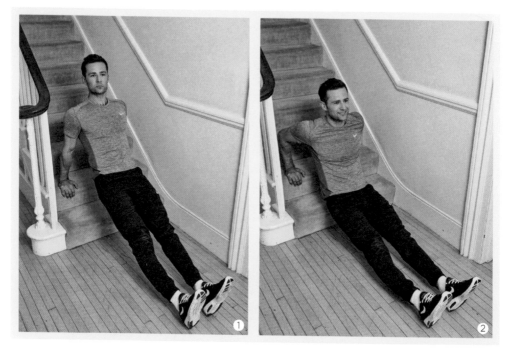

Jump squat

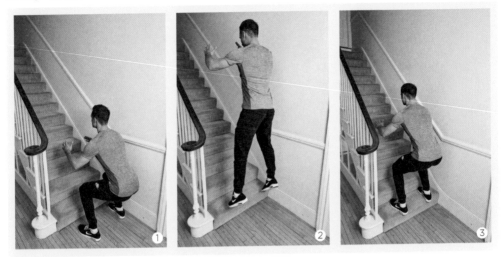

Split lunge (left leg)

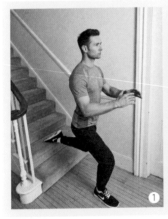

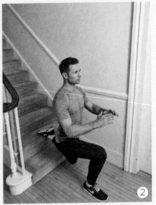

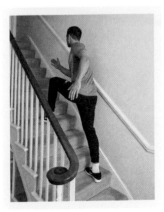

Run up the stairs – three steps at a time.

IF YOU CAN'T STAND THE HEAT...

—

You'll need a tea towel, some bottles of water, some tins of baked beans and some cookbooks for this workout – I recommend Delia Smith's Complete Cookery Course if you're doing the advanced workout! I did promise exercise can be done anywhere, using anything ...

For a five-minute workout repeat each of these exercises for one minute. To increase it to a ten-minute workout try adding one of the extra moves from pages 132-133 in between each of the exercises in the workout. If you want to really feel the burn, add some spice and do two rounds for a 20-minute workout.

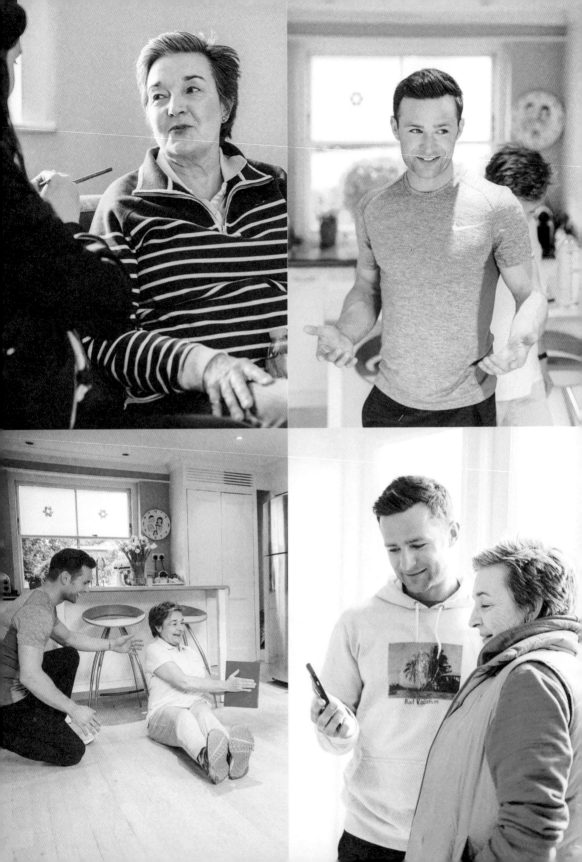

Push-up – off the table or worktop.

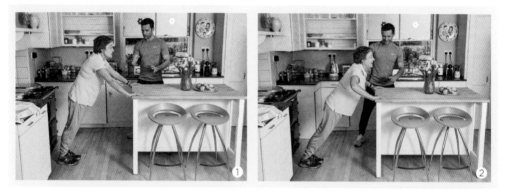

Single leg tuck – use a tea towel to allow for slide. You can work out and clean at the same time here: bonus!

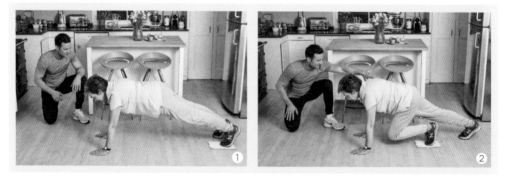

Cookbook twist – keep your feet on the floor and use one cookbook to start with.

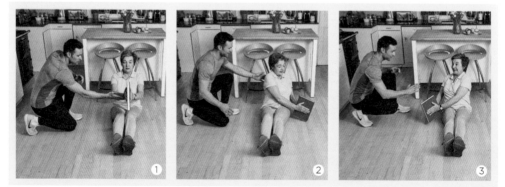

Single arm reverse fly – use a tin of baked beans (or similar) to add some weight.

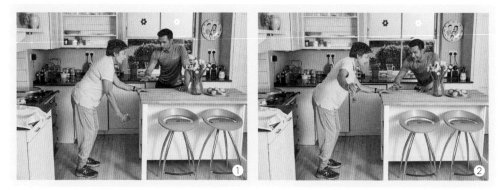

Breakfast stool dip – you could use a chair, bench or whatever you've got.

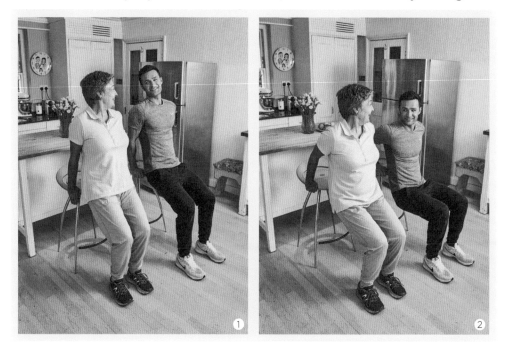

INTERMEDIATE

Push-up – knees on the floor.

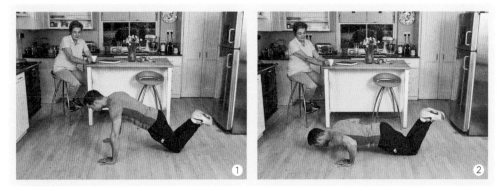

Knee tuck

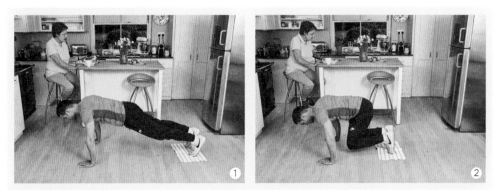

Cookbook twist – use two books and try with your feet in the air.

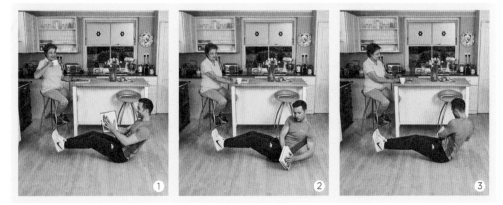

Single arm reverse fly – knees on the floor. Try using a full water bottle (you can drink it after your workout is complete!)

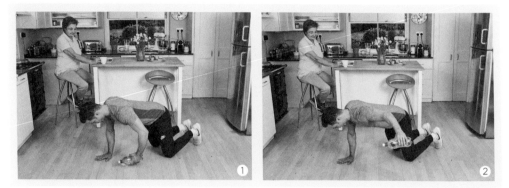

Breakfast stool dip – straighten your legs.

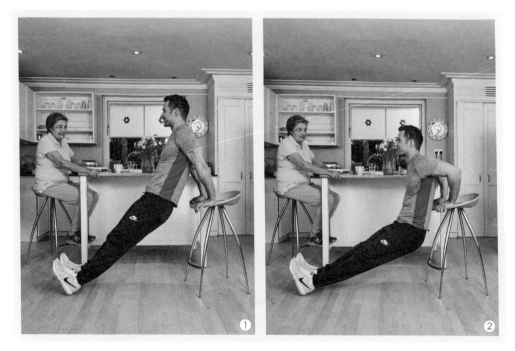

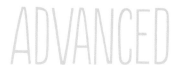

Cookbook push-up – slide the book forward on the way down. Alternate each arm.

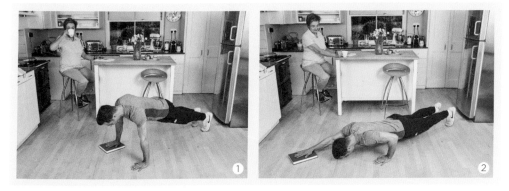

Single leg tuck – keep one leg in the air whilst you tuck the other in.

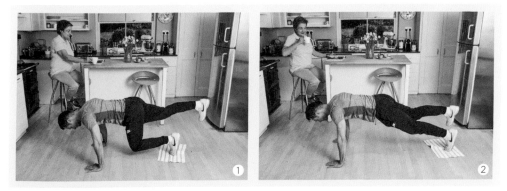

Cookbook twist – use three books.

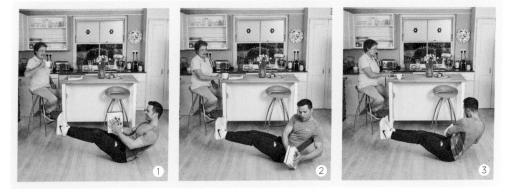

Single arm reverse fly – use a large full bottle of water.

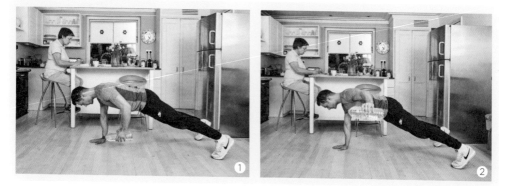

Breakfast bar dip

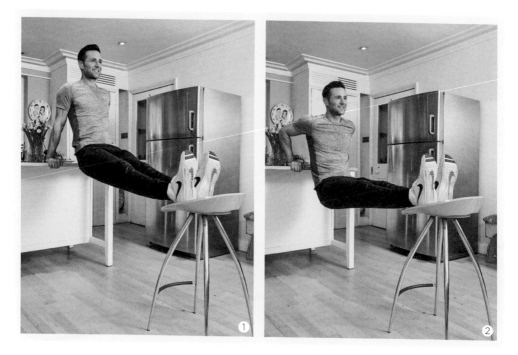

ADDITIONAL EXERCISES

Add these exercises in between each exercise in the workout to increase the length of your workout to ten minutes. For beginners perform each exercise for 40 seconds, rest for 20 seconds. At intermediate level perform each exercise for 50 seconds with a 10 second rest and for advanced ability perform each exercise for one minute with no rest.

Squat and front raise – water bottles are optional but the bigger the bottle, the harder it is.

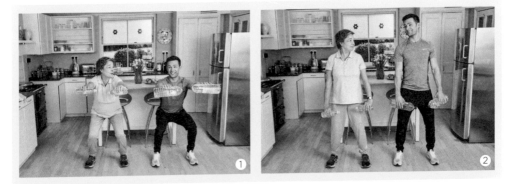

Lunge and side raise

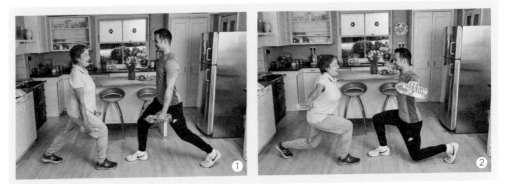

Cookbook sliding reverse lunge – focus on a smooth reverse slide.

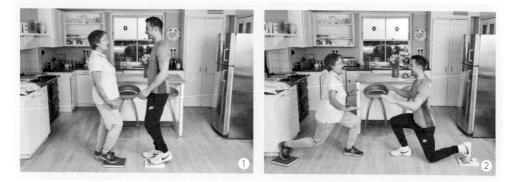

Cookbook sliding adductor – squeeze your inner thigh on the way back.

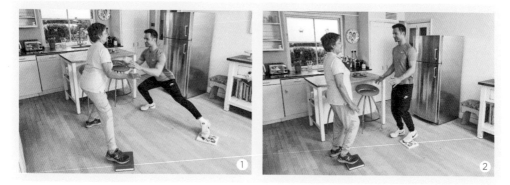

Deadlift – the more cookbooks, the harder the lift. Keep your core engaged and a slight bend in your knees.

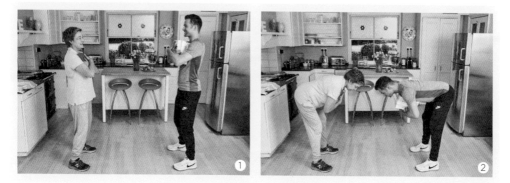

THE DAILY
COMMUTE

—

Going for a run or walk is a really good way to get in some exercise, but I also find it is one of the best ways to clear my head. Maybe you can try swapping a bus journey to work with a run instead. I like to mix up my running sometimes by throwing in some body weight exercises. For example, you could try running for five minutes then stopping to do one of these exercises for a minute, run for another five minutes before trying another exercise and so on...

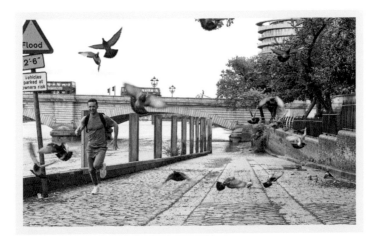

Push-up

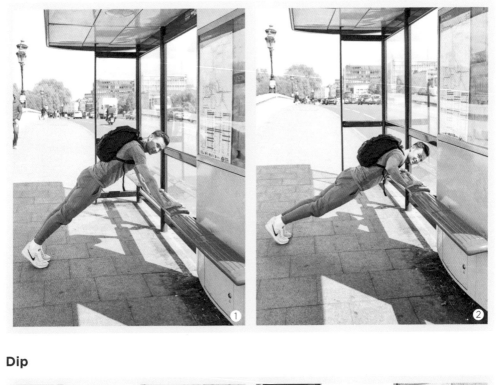

Dip

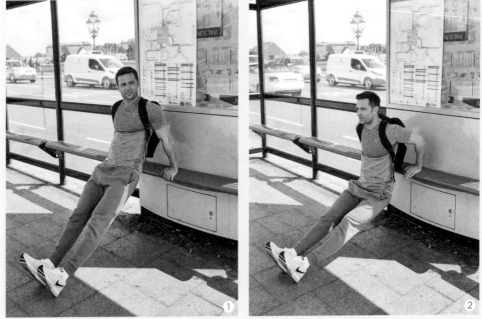

Leg raise – now clearly I don't expect you to do this at the bus stop, you can try finding a solid looking branch on a tree in a park.

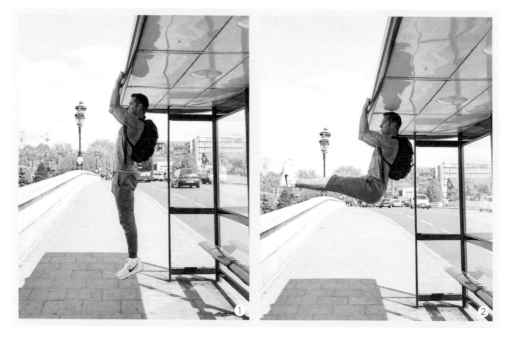

Pull-up – why did the chicken cross the road? To do some pull-ups.

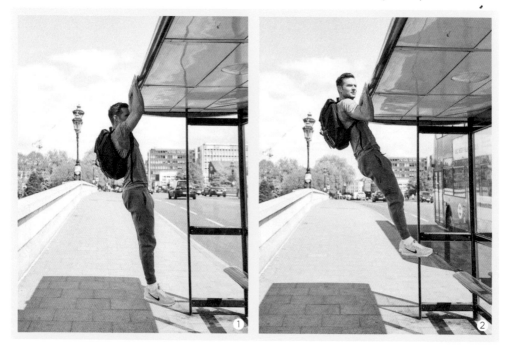

Split squat

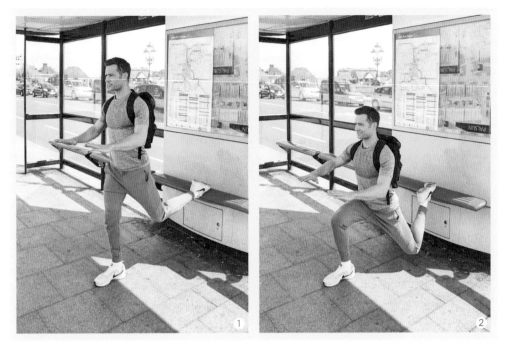

These exercises are pretty advanced. You could just as easily try:

- SQUATS OR SQUAT JUMPS

- BURPEES

- PUSH-UPS

- SOME CORE EXERCISES FROM PAGES 214–217.

HARRY'S DESKERCISE

You couldn't call my job an office job, but more and more is being discovered about the negative effects of sitting for long periods of time each day (see page 78). Everyone I've tried this out on agrees that a bit of exercise makes you more productive at work and positive about the hours ahead. Exercising in the day before a show certainly helps my performance in a gig.

Do each of the five exercises for one minute to make a five-minute workout. Repeat for a longer ten-minute session.

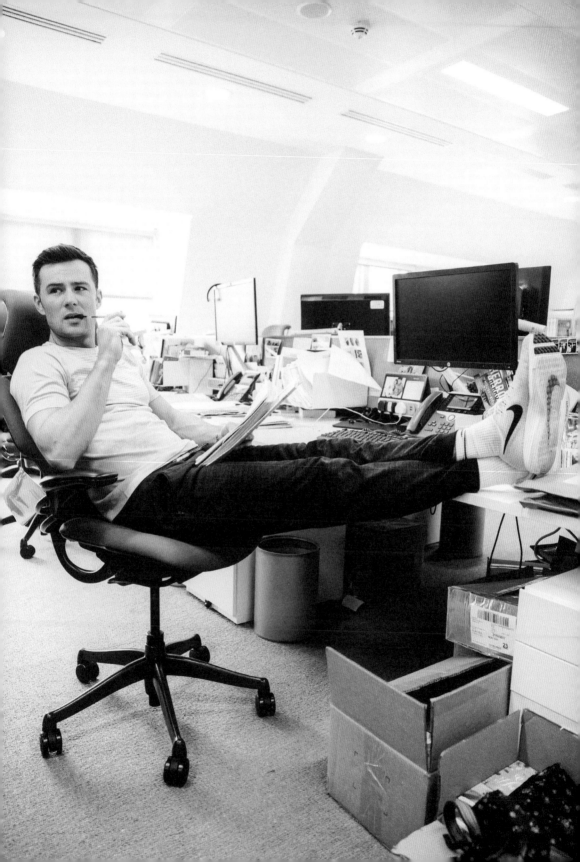

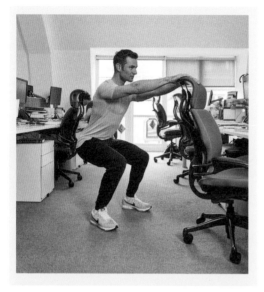

Chair squat – squat whilst holding the chair for balance.

Desk push-up

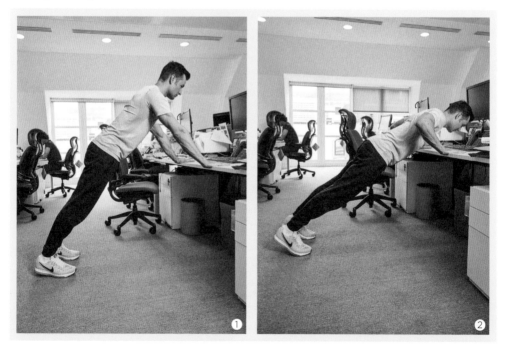

Lunge – hold your chair to help you balance.

Straight arm plank

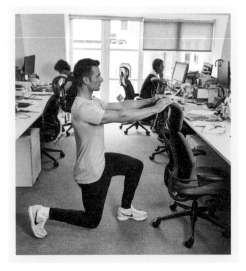
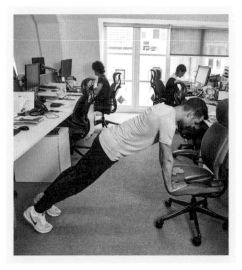

Desk dip – keep your legs bent. Worried about your colleagues thinking you look weird? Get them to join in!

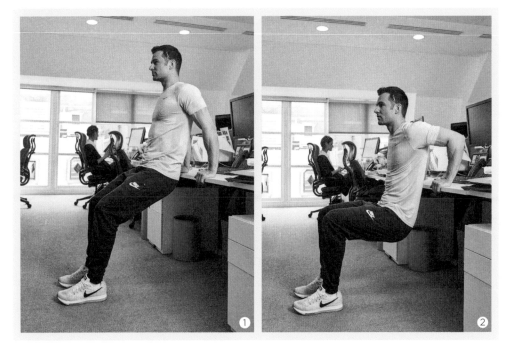

INTERMEDIATE

Squat

Push-up on your knees

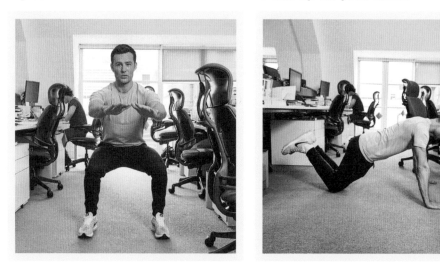

Static lunge – 25 seconds each leg.

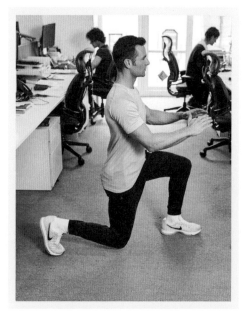

Chair rollout – put your knees on the floor and push out with your arms. Make sure you use a chair with wheels!

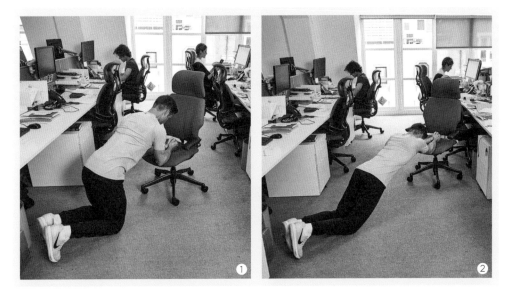

Chair dip – bent or straight legs.

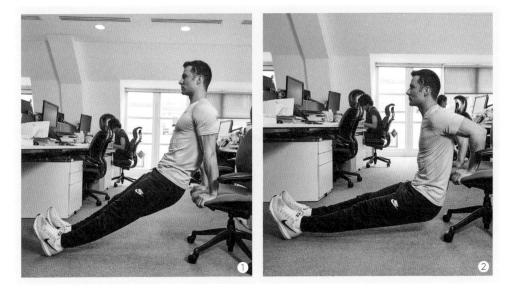

ADVANCED

Chair split squat

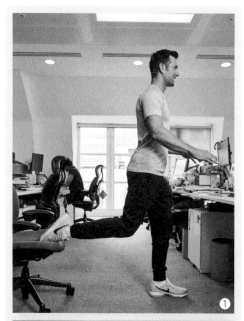

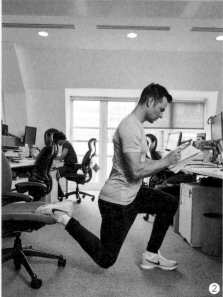

Decline push-up and knee – once
you've completed the push-up, roll
the chair in by tucking your knees in!

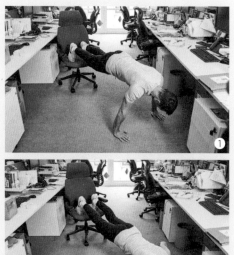

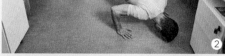

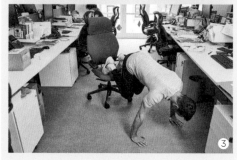

Pistol squat – holding the desk or seat is optional.

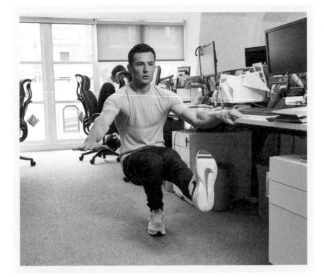

Straight-arm rollout

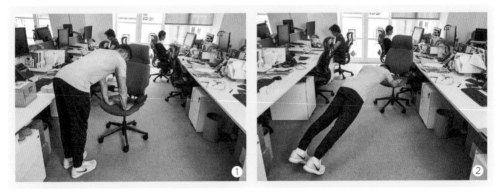

Dip – with your feet on the chair

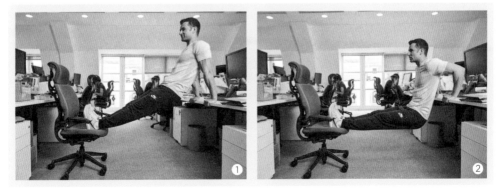

OFFICE AEROBICS

Don't fancy doing deskercise on your own? Get a group together and try some of these in your lunch break. Perform each exercise for 30 seconds with no rest inbetween to get a quick five minute group workout. Repeat as many times as you like!

Jogging on the spot – then reach your arms out and up and repeat.

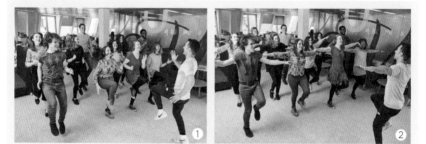

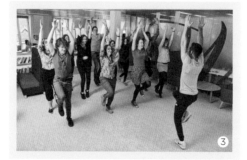

Single leg knee raise – bring a knee up to the opposite elbow. Alternate.

Hand to opposite foot – alternate.

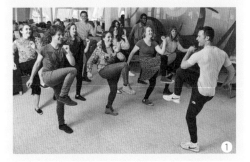

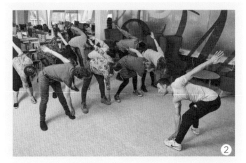

Jumping Jacks – stand with your feet together and hands at your sides. Simultaneously raise your arms above your head and jump out spreading your feet wide. Quickly reverse the movement and repeat.

Spotty Dogs – jump landing with one foot forward and the other back whilst raising the opposite arm to your forward leg.

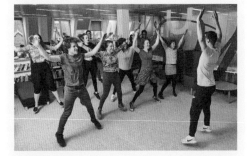

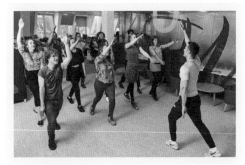

Burpee

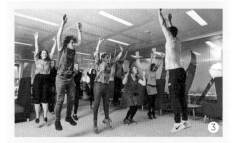

Crunch

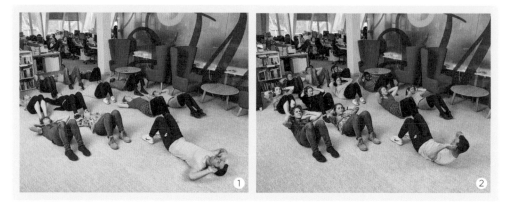

Straight arm plank – whilst planking, tuck one knee in then extend out. Alternate.

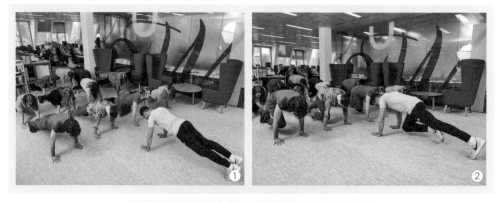

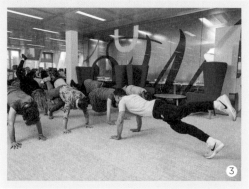

Squat – pair up and high five at the top of the squat, or a high ten if you're feeling crazy.

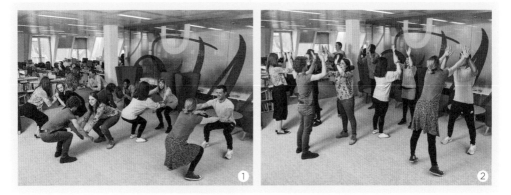

Push-up – with a low five at the top of the push-up.

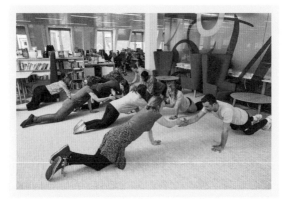

Sprint on and off – five seconds on, five seconds off for the 30 seconds.

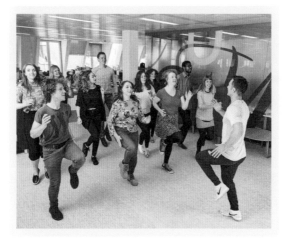

HITTING THE

WALL

—

All you need is a wall. Indoors, outdoors … it doesn't matter. Between you and a wall you can get a really good workout in. If you're at my house, no shoes and make sure your hands are clean first (did somebody say OCD?)!

Take one minute per exercise for a ten-minute workout and you'll feel good after it I'm sure.

—

Wall walk – keep your hands in the same place and walk your feet up and down the wall.

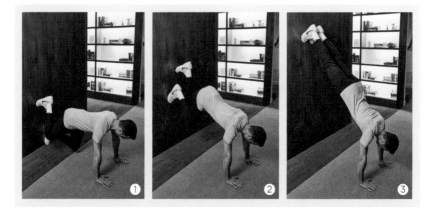

Wall squat – hold this for a minute, think happy thoughts.

Handstand

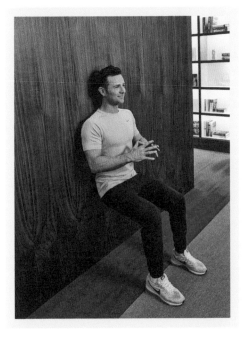

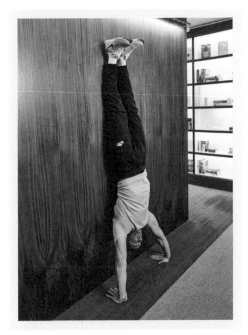

Handstand press – be warned this is tough!

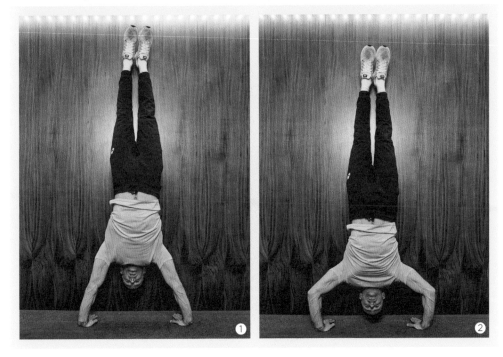

Wall walk with hands – not advised for those with clammy hands.

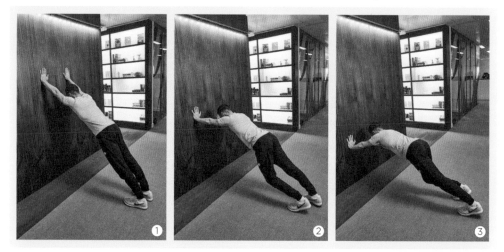

Wall push-up

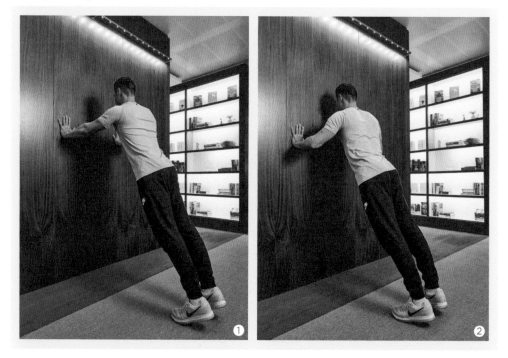

Pistol squat – slide down the wall and drive back up through your leg.

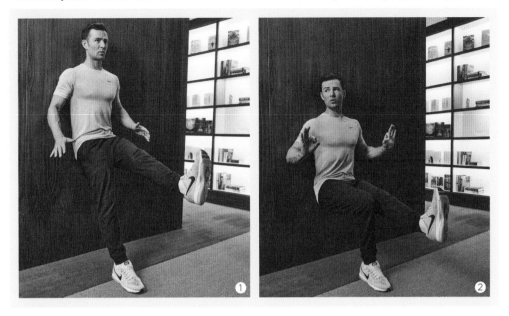

Glute bridge – both legs or single leg.

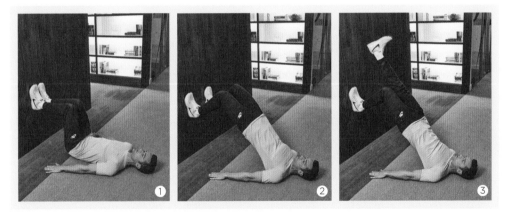

Wall plank – from plank position place hands on the wall one at a time and then back to the floor.

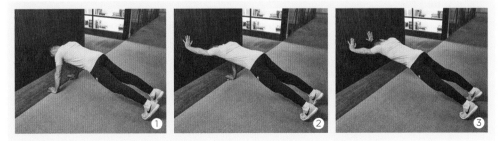

HOW MUCH CAN YOU (PARK) BENCH?

Don't worry, I'm not going to ask you to lift a park bench. But you can use it to make an awesome workout. I love training outside when the weather's good, but I've been known to do it in the rain and snow too (makes me feel like Rocky Balboa in Rocky IV!).

Once again, if you keep repeating each exercise until you hit a minute and then move on, by the time you have done them all you'll have done a great five-minute workout. If you fancy making it a bit longer though, in between each of the exercises, do a 50-100 metre sprint and then walk back.

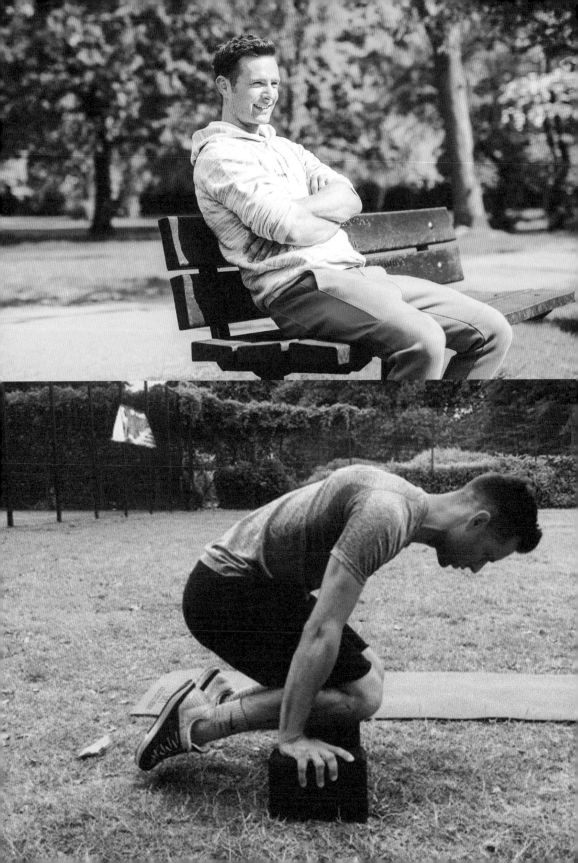

Bench sit squat – sit down at the bottom
of the squat and stand back up.

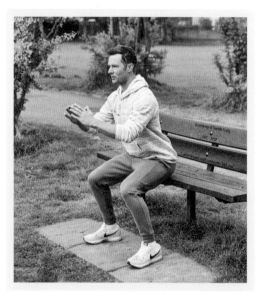

Push-up – use the back of the bench.

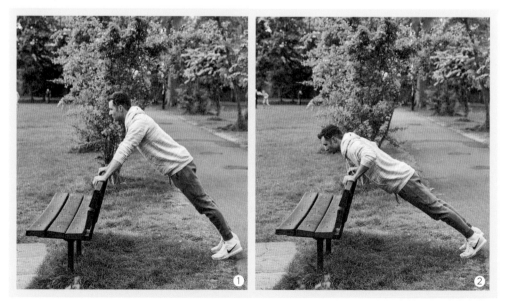

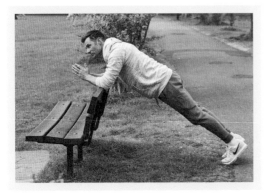

Plank – you'll be resting your forearms on the back of the bench so use something to cushion your arms.

Step-up – step up, raise opposite knee up and then step down so both feet are back on the floor. Do 25 seconds on each leg then swap.

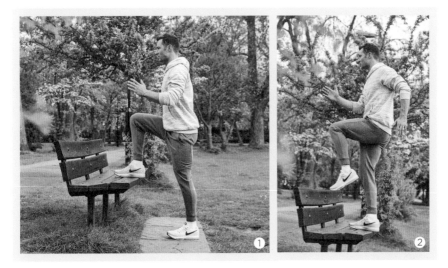

Dip – use the back of the bench.

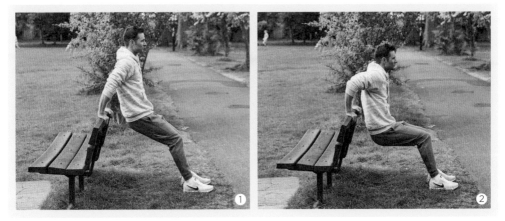

INTERMEDIATE

Perform each exercise for 50 seconds, rest for 10 seconds.

Squat – tap your bum on the seat.

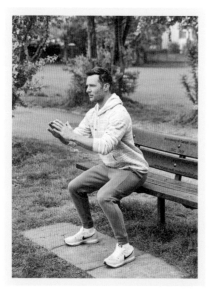

Push-up – with hands on the seat.

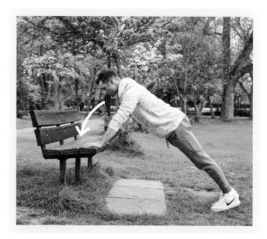

Step-up – step up, raise opposite knee up and then step down so both feet are back on the floor. Do 25 seconds on each leg then swap.

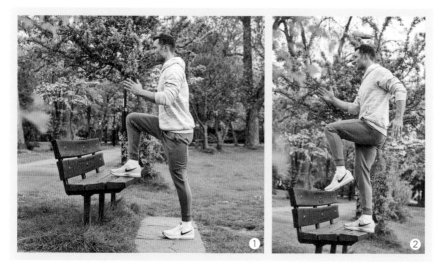

Plank

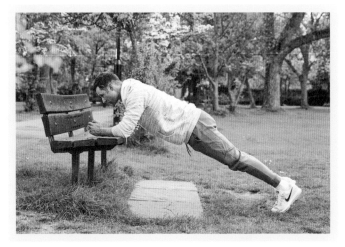

Dip – legs bent or straight.

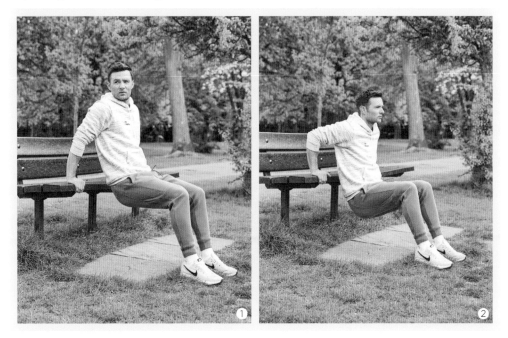

ADVANCED

Split squat – make it harder by adding a jump. 30 seconds on each leg.

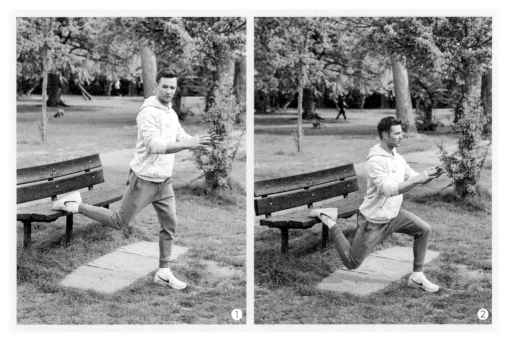

Decline push-up

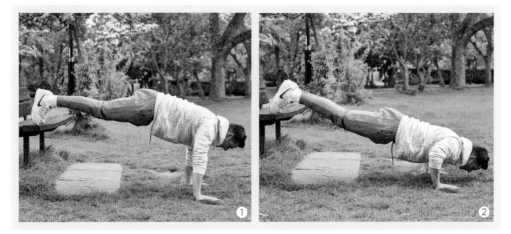

Step-up – with a jump at the top.

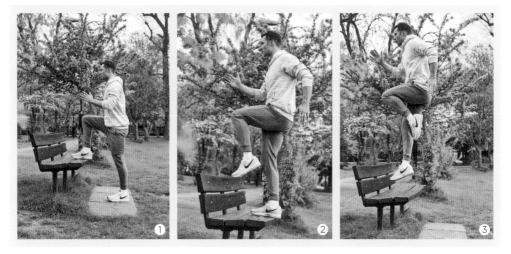

Plank – tap the bench with alternating hands. Keep as steady as possible.

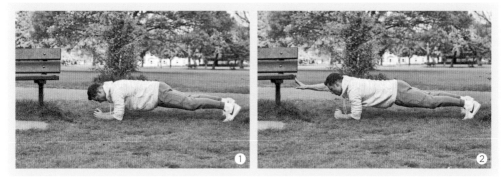

Dip

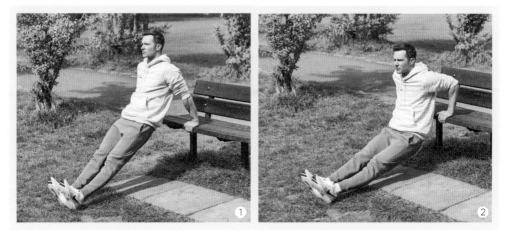

BODYWEIGHT WITH A MATE

—

I love exercising with friends. It spurs me on to work harder. (Competitive? Who, me?) It's a good chance to catch up as well as doing something productive. I often get the giggles when I'm exercising with mates, but that's fine – when you're laughing and out of breath it makes it a bit more of a challenge. And laughing's a good core exercise, too!

  This one is a ten-minute workout.

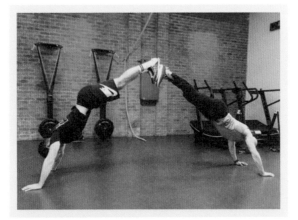

Squat and dip – the person squatting can use a wall or tree. The person performing the dip can have their legs bent or straight for a tougher workout.

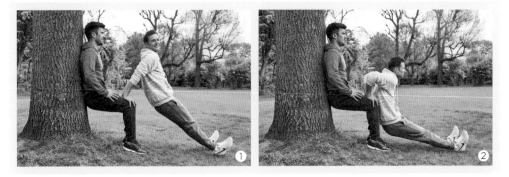

Decline push-up and squat – each person goes down into their exercise at the same time.

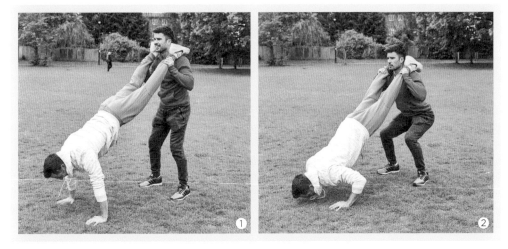

Assisted pistol squat – this one is tough so good luck!

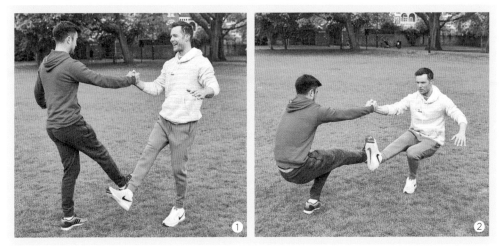

Resisted shoulder press – the person standing pushes down to provide resistance.

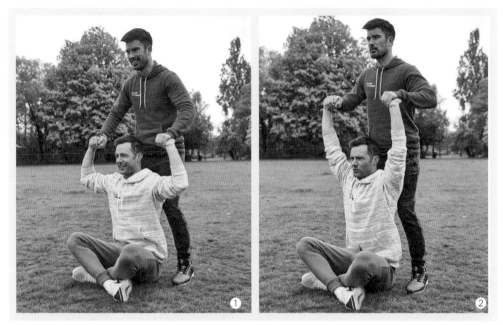

Plank arm wrestle – may the best person win!

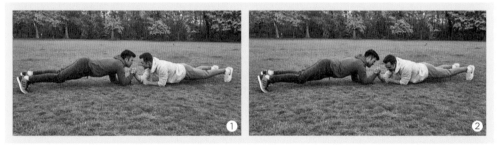

Bent over row – positioning is key for the person standing: keep your core engaged.

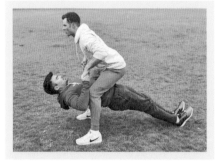

Static squat – back to back: who can last the longest?!

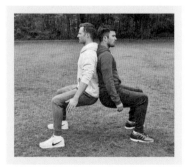

Push and pull – holding hands try pushing with one hand and pull with the other then swap.

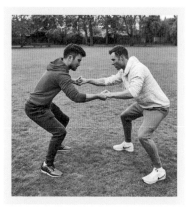

Push-up – an advanced move with your partner on your back.

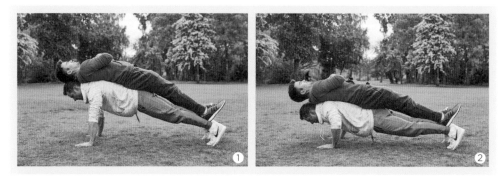

Push-up – Do a high five at the top of the push-up. Don't forget to alternate hands.

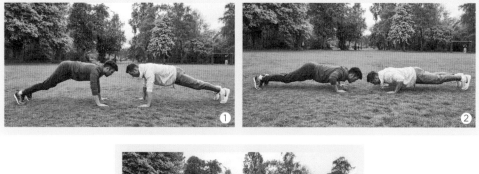

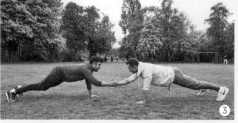

HARRY'S HEROES

I gave this workout this title because it's a super-challenging 12-minute session – I find it tough to complete the advanced level of this, so if you manage any of them, you're a bit of a hero.

   I've included some suggestions for times but you can mix this up – feel free to play around with timing, you know how hard you need to work.

Walk > jog > sprint x 2

BEGINNERS:
10 secs walk, 10 secs jog, 10 secs sprint, 1 min rest. Repeat.

INTERMEDIATE:
20 secs walk, 20 secs jog, 20 secs sprint, 30 secs rest. Repeat.

ADVANCED:
30 secs walk, 30 secs jog, 30 secs sprint, no rest. Repeat.

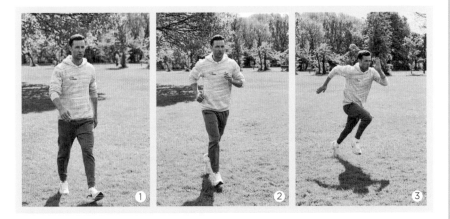

Squats or squat jumps

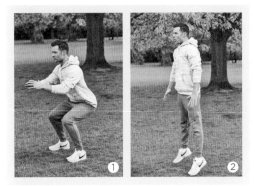

BEGINNERS:
Squat for 30 secs, rest for 30 secs.

INTERMEDIATE:
Squat jumps for 30 secs, rest for 30 secs.

ADVANCED:
Squat jumps for 1 min, no rest.

Walk > jog > sprint x 2 – as before

Push-ups

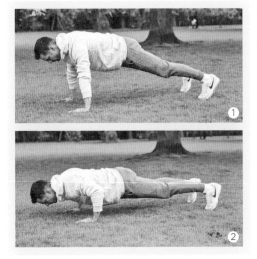

BEGINNERS:
Push-ups off a tree for 30 secs, rest for 30 secs.

INTERMEDIATE:
Push-ups on your knees for 40secs, rest for 20 secs.

ADVANCED:
Push-ups for 1 full minute, no rest.

Walk > jog > sprint x 2 – as before

Burpees

BEGINNERS:	INTERMEDIATE:	ADVANCED:
no jump	with jump	chest to the floor

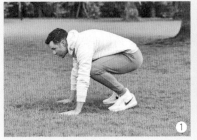
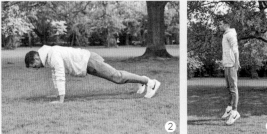

HIT THE BAR

No, not that bar, I'm afraid. Being a non-drinker, this
is the kind of bar I'm most interested in these days.
 These are great strength exercises that I like to do
in the park. These are certainly advanced exercises.
I recommend you pick two or three of these exercises.
Perform however many reps feels suitable to you and
do three rounds. Mix it up and try different variations.

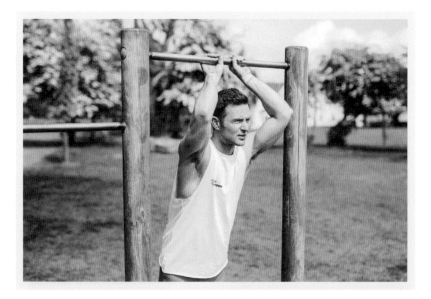

Pull-ups – keep your core engaged. If you are just starting out then try jumping into position 2 and slowly let yourself down.

Wide grip

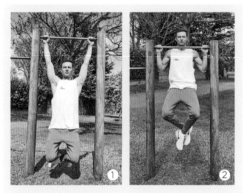

Close grip

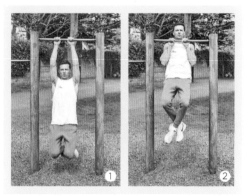

Reverse grip

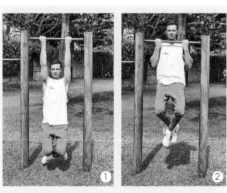

L-sit

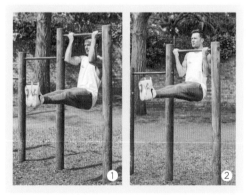

Leg raise– engage your back, arms and core and keep your legs as straight as possible.

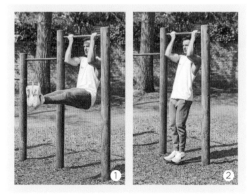

Knee tuck

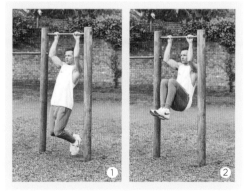

Windscreen wipers – the wipers on the bus go swish, swish, swish... !

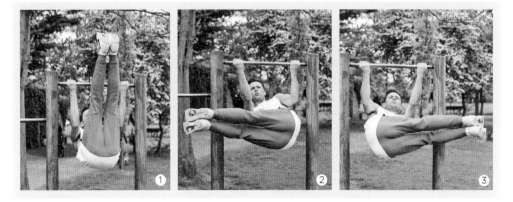

Bar row – dig your heels in. The further away your feet are, the harder it becomes.

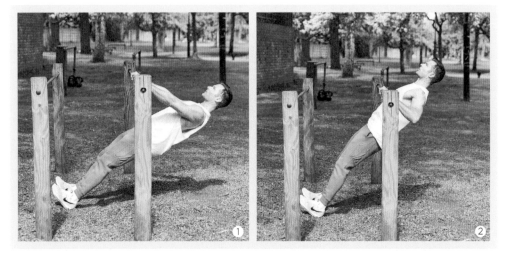

Ab rollout – using a swing.

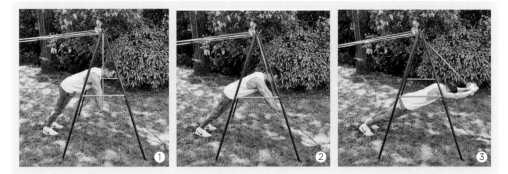

Push-up and knee tuck – do the push-up then tuck your knees in.

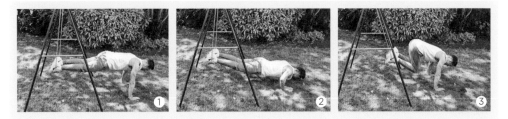

Handstand press – once in the handstand position, lower yourself down and push yourself back up. If, unlike me, you're really hardcore you won't even need a wall.

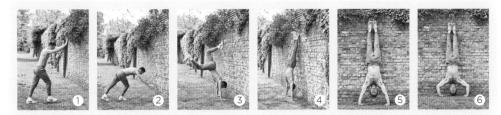

Slide hop

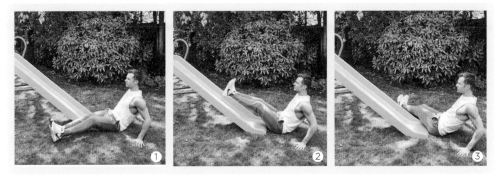

Slide V-sit

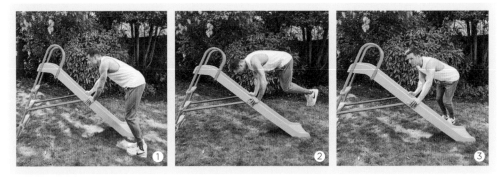

GARDEN

—

Another outdoor workout, but you don't need a huge garden (mine's tiny), just a little bit of outside space. My mum particularly enjoys this workout – she found it achievable and a good starting point.

For a five-minute workout repeat each of these exercises for one minute. To increase it to a ten-minute workout try adding the core moves on page 179 in between each of the exercises. If you want to really feel the burn, do two rounds for a 20-minute workout.

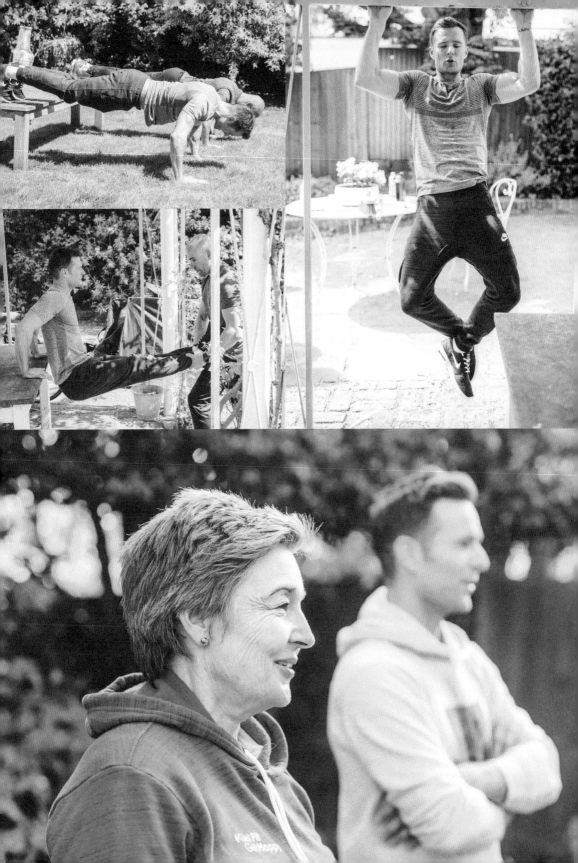

Sun salutation – start with a slight bend in the knees and straighten your legs when your arms are at the top.

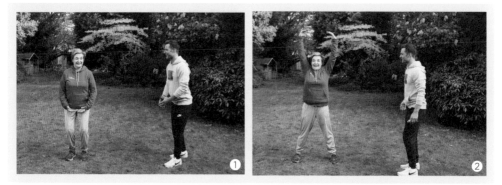

Upper body rotation – step slightly as you rotate your upper body.

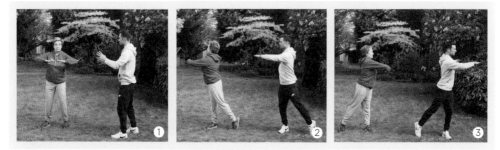

Jog on the spot

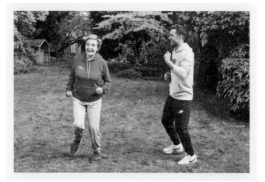

Star jump

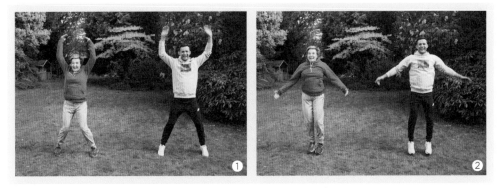

Back and forth – find a starting and end point and then jog forwards to the end point, and then backwards to the starting point. Repeat.

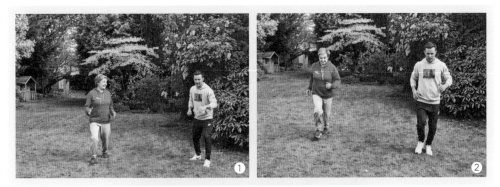

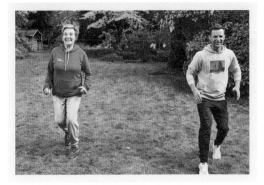

INTERMEDIATE

Perform each exercise for 50 seconds, rest for 10 seconds.

Sun salutation and squat

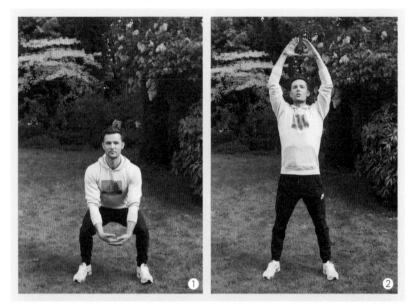

Side skater – jumping side to side as if you are ice skating.

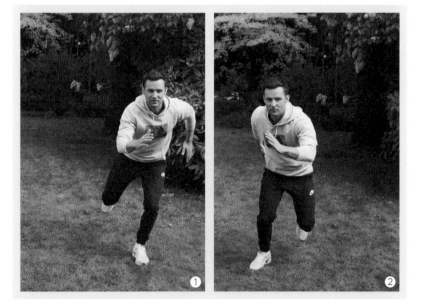

Run on the spot

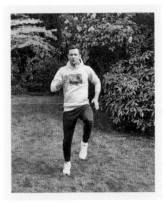

Star jump

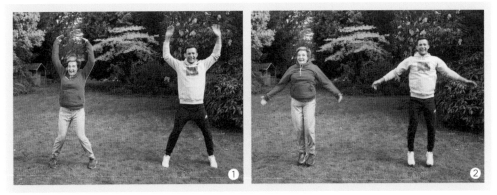

Back and forth – find a starting and end point and run forwards towards the end point and touch the floor, then run back toward the starting point. Repeat.

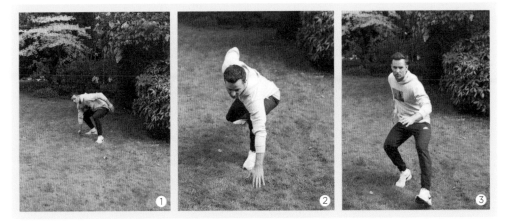

ADVANCED

Sun salutation with jump squat

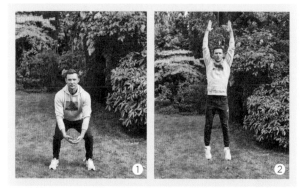

Single leg plyo lateral squat – side skaters with greater depth and distance.

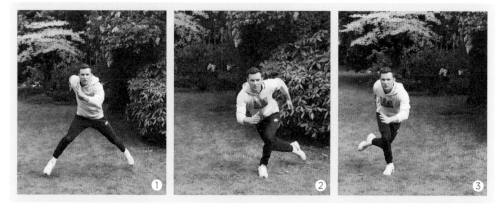

Sprint on the spot

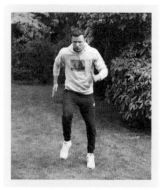

Explosive star jump – hands to feet.

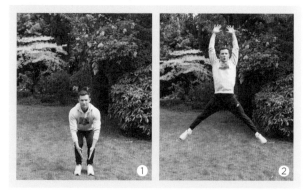

Back and forth – find a starting and end point and sprint forwards towards the end point and touch the floor, then run backwards toward the starting point. Repeat.

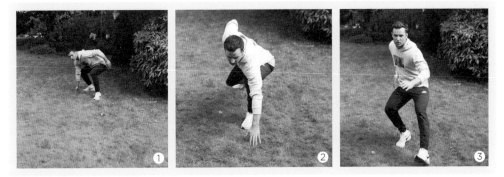

CORE EXERCISES

Use the same work and rest timings as throughout your workout according to ability.

Crunch

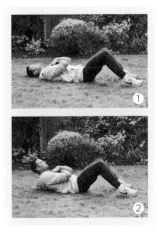

Dorsal raise

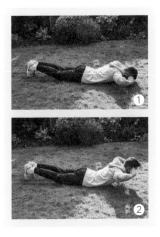

Plank with leg raise – raise one leg up and then alternate.

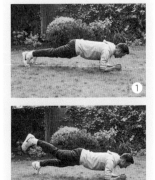

Knee tap – touch knee with opposite hand. Alternate.

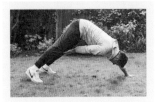

Toe tap – touch toe with opposite hand. Alternate.

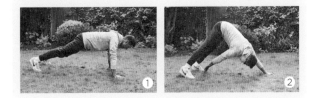

HAIR OF THE DOG

We've all been there, and it's not fun! But honestly, when I was hungover, I used to recover by doing some exercise and it always made me feel better. Another important thing when you're hanging is to drink plenty of fluids, so in this workout you won't just be sweating it out, you'll be rehydrating too. You'll need five glasses or bottles of water laid out in a line. If you're really hanging, ignore the 'x 2' part!

Run – between glasses or bottles of water, there and back, facing forwards x 2

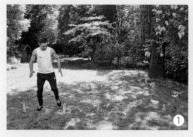
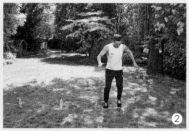

Air punches – 10 punches in front of each glass, there and back.

Drink the first glass of water.

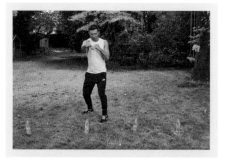
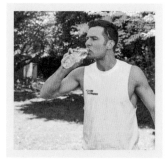

Side jumps – to each glass, there and back.

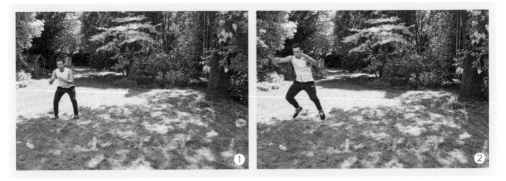

Push-ups – do as many as you like at each glass, there and back.

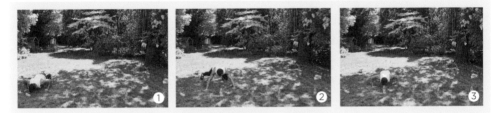

Drink the second glass of water.

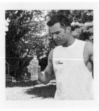

Burpees – do a burpee at each glass, there and back.

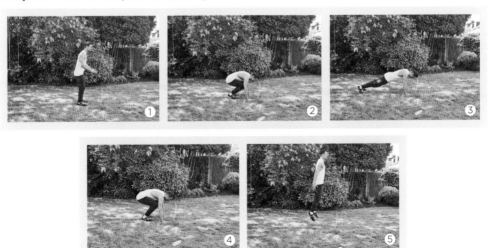

Inch worm – at each glass, there and back. Get into starting position and whilst keeping your feet still, walk forwards with your hands until you are in position 3 and then walk back up to standing position.

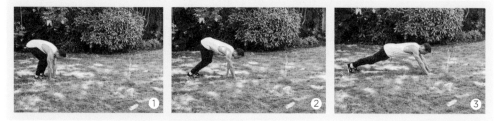

Drink the third glass of water.

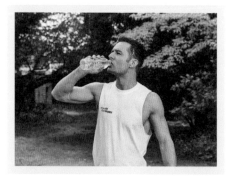

Slalom run – between glasses, there and back x 2.

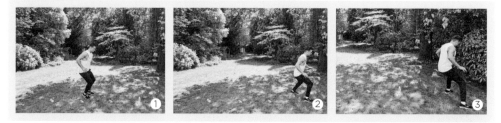

Squat jump – over glasses, there and back x 2.

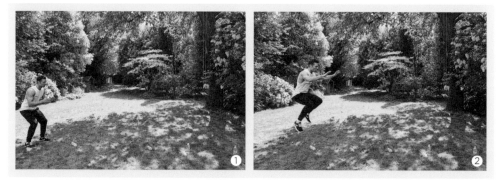

Drink the fourth glass of water.

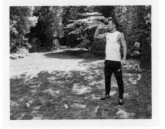

High knees– do 10 reps at each glass, there and back.

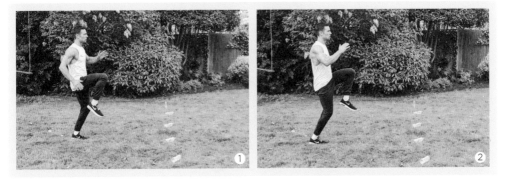

Mountain climbers – do 10 reps at each glass, there and back.

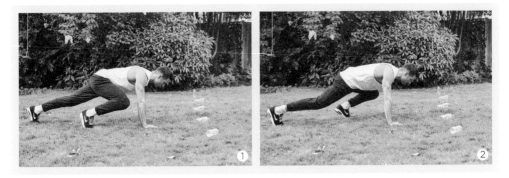

Drink the fifth glass of water.

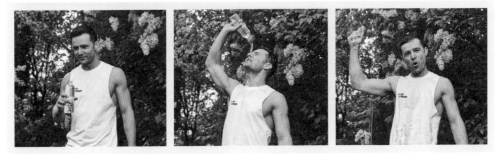

LOUNGING AROUND

This is one for the sitting room – but you're not going to be doing any sitting (feel free to have the TV on though). Use a chair or a sofa to help you perform the exercises. Managed it? Sofa so good ...

   This is another of those five-minute workouts that you can take up to ten minutes by adding in one of the cardio exercises from pages 190-191 in between each of the excercises in the workout. Push it that bit further and do two rounds to make it up to 20 minutes.

BEGINNER
Perform each exercise for 40 seconds, rest for 20 seconds.

Push-up – use the back of the chair or sofa.

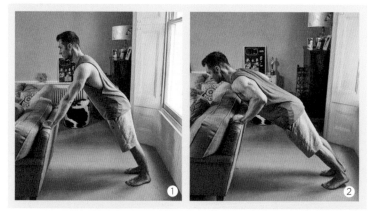

Assisted squat – use a chair or sofa for balance.

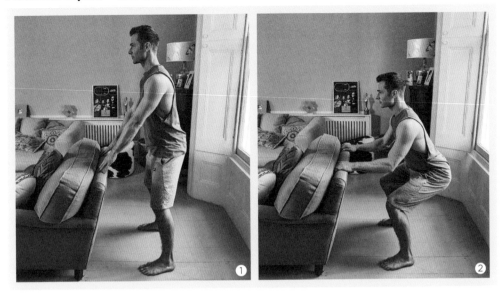

Dip

Plank

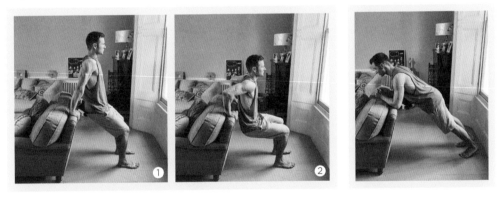

Bridge – position your feet wide.

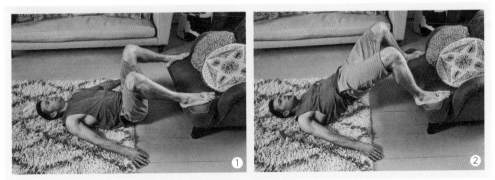

INTERMEDIATE

Perform each exercise for 50 seconds, rest for 10 seconds.

Push-up

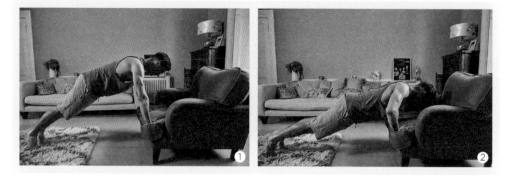

Bum tap squat

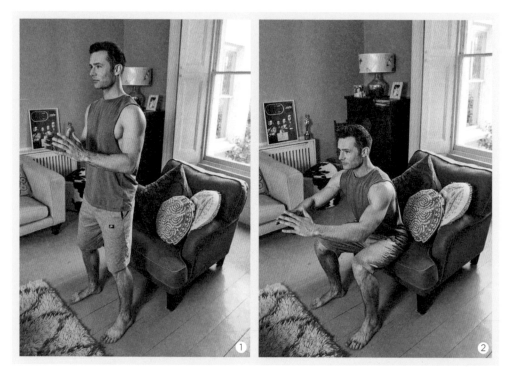

Plank

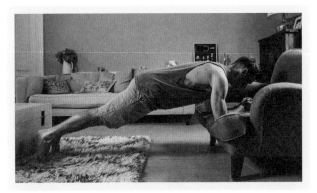

Dip

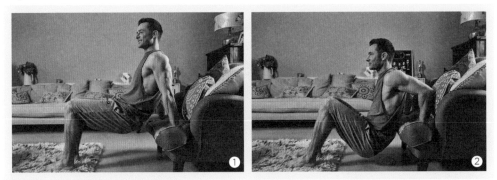

Bridge – position your feet close.

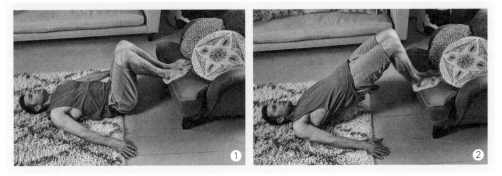

ADVANCED

Perform each exercise for one minute, no rest.

Decline push-up

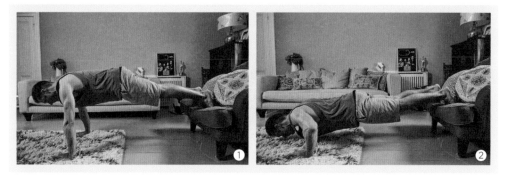

Pistol squat –holding a chair or sofa for balance if required.

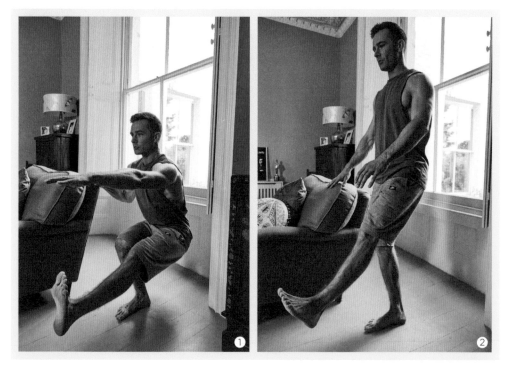

Dip – rest your feet on the coffee table and keep your legs straight.

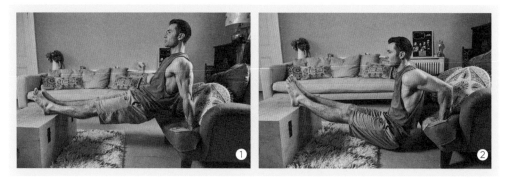

Plank – with alternating chair or sofa tap

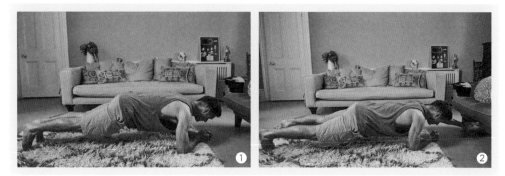

Single leg bridge

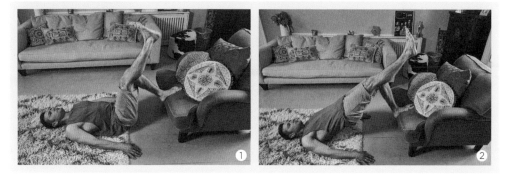

ADDITIONAL CARDIO EXERCISES

Add these five cardio moves in between each strength exercise to increase the length of your workout to ten minutes. For beginners perform each exercise for 40 seconds, rest for 20 seconds. At intermediate level perform each exercise for 50 seconds with 10 seconds rest and for advanced level perform each exercise for one minute with no rest.

Foot tap – on the chair or sofa   **Jumping Jacks**

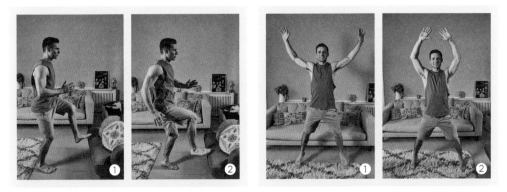

Mountain climbers – the chair is optional, you could just do this on the floor!

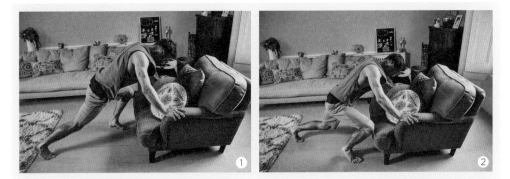

Spotty dogs

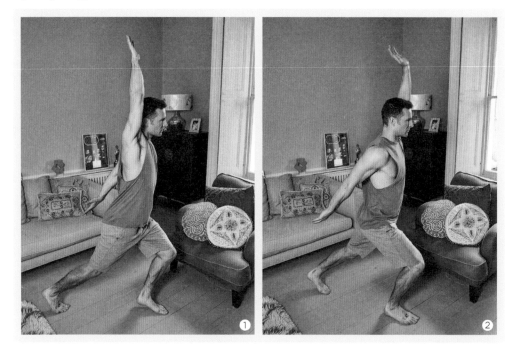

Hop-over

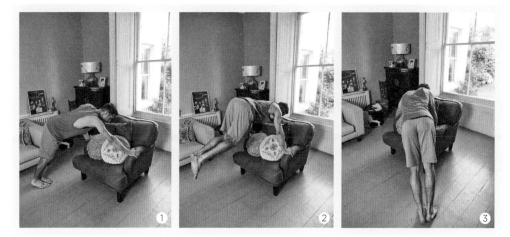

SELFIE WORKOUT

Everyone loves a selfie, so why not incorporate it into your exercise? Take a selfie after each individual exercise. I'm hoping that your photos will become less and less flattering. You'll be smiling by the end (kind of!), I promise. Bang it over to me on Instagram with the hashtags #getfitgethappy and #selfieworkout for a double tap.

Repeat each exercise as many times as you can in 20 seconds and then take 10 seconds to take that all-important selfie. If the selfies are still looking too flattering, ramp it up a bit more, repeat each exercise for 50 seconds and then have that 10-second selfie break before you move onto the next one.

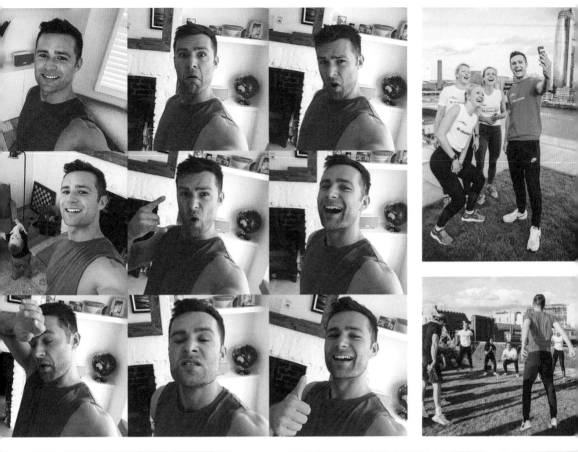
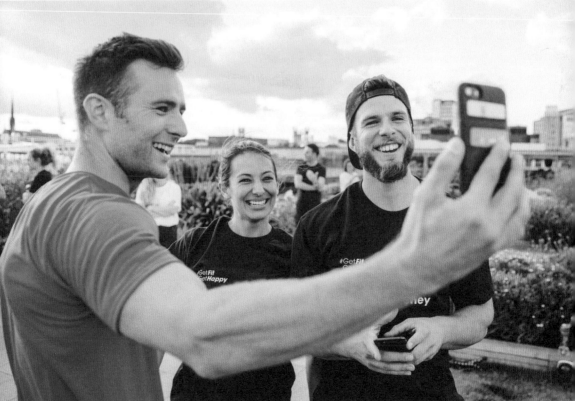

Squat – or jump squat.

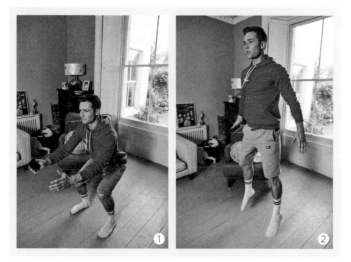

Mountain climbers – use a chair or do this on the floor to make it harder if you prefer.

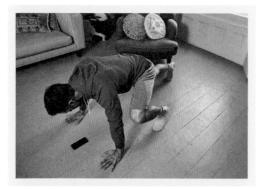

Left leg lunge – or alternating jump lunges (as shown).

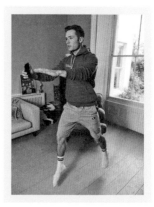

Knees to floor push-up – or normal push-up to make it harder.

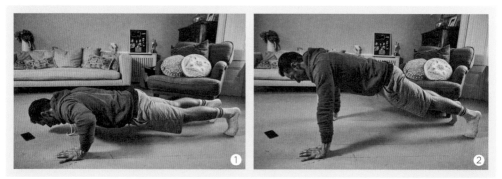

Right leg lunge (shown) – or alternating jump lunges.

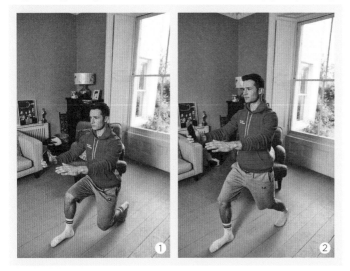

Plank

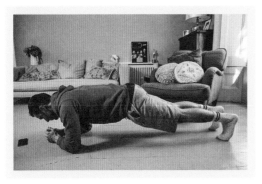

High knees

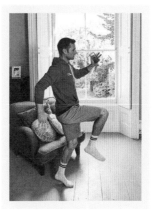

Side hop – use a chair or on the floor.

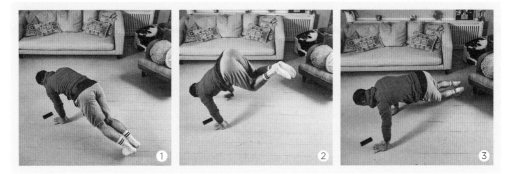

HAPPY

WORKOUT

——

I put this together alongside the song 'Happy' by Pharrell Williams. Every time you hear the word 'happy' you're going to have to perform a move and you'll soon realise just how many times 'happy' appears in the song. Feel free to use the pause button! But the challenge is to try to complete the full song. Good luck.

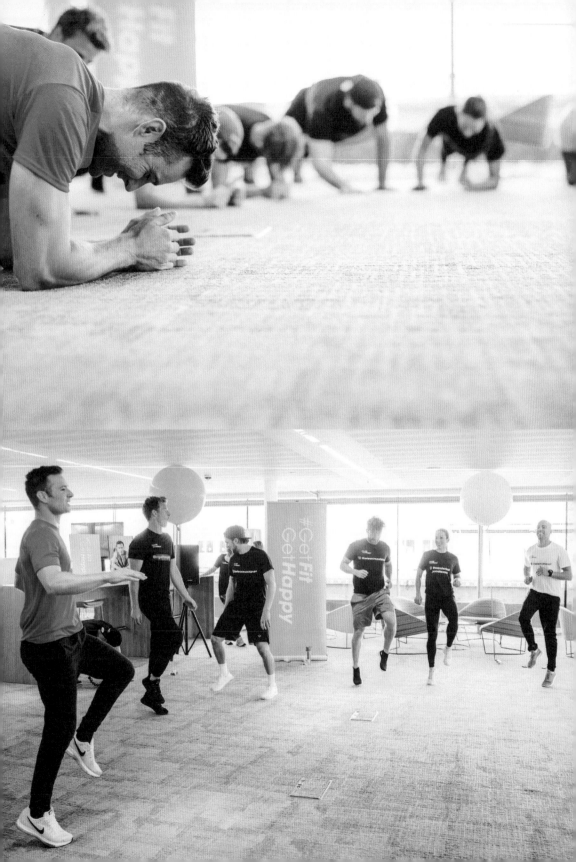

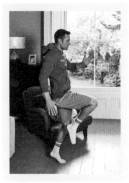

High knees to the beat

Chorus 1: Continue with high knees to the beat but every time you hear the word 'happy' in the backing vocals do a burpee.

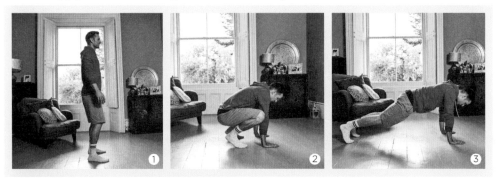

Verse 2: Plank – stay in the plank position for the duration of the verse.

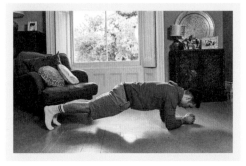

Chorus 2: Continue planking and add in a push-up on every 'happy'.

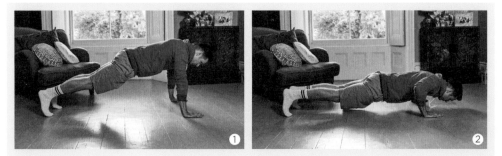

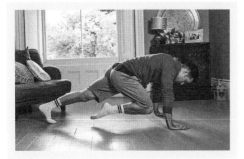

Mountain climbers to the beat

Chorus 3: Continue with high knees to the beat but every time you hear the word 'happy' in the backing vocals do a burpee.

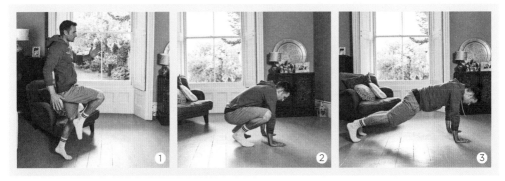

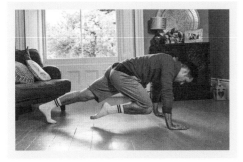

Bridge 2 (clapping section):
Mountain climbers to the beat

Chorus 4: Plank throughout the chorus and perform a push-up on every 'happy'.

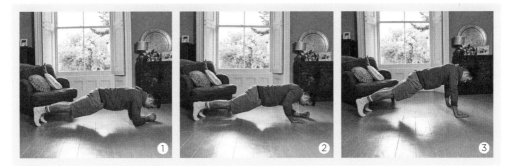

SOCK IT TO YOU

All you need is two pairs of (clean!) socks. I know it sounds weird but stick with me – this one's pretty tough. It requires some strength and determination. I personally love this workout because I enjoy doing strength work. You can't do this on the carpet – you'll need a smooth floor. Ten exercises, ten minutes: away you go!

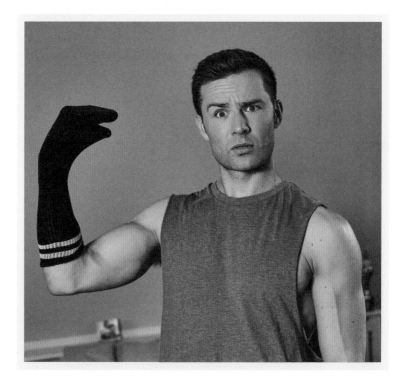

SOCKS ON FEET

Push-up with a double knee tuck

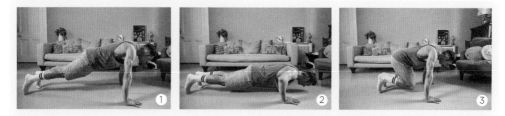

Mountain slider – like a mountain climber but slide your feet on the floor.

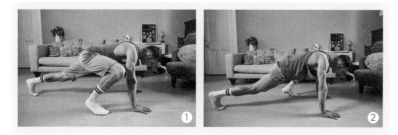

Glute bridge slider – slide your feet into the bridge position and squeeze those glutes!

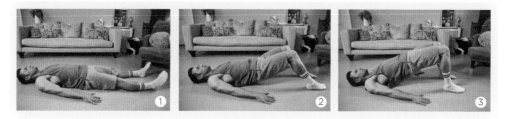

Pike – keep your hands stationary and slide your feet into a pike (position 2) and then slide them back.

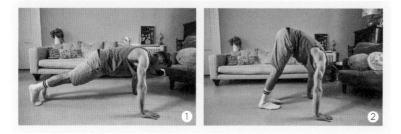

Dragging yourself forward – keep your feet and legs in the same position and while moving your hands forward drag away!

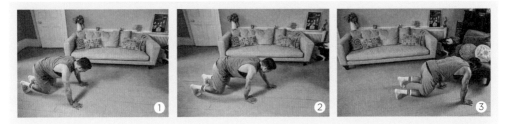

Windscreen wipers – slide your legs out and then back in.

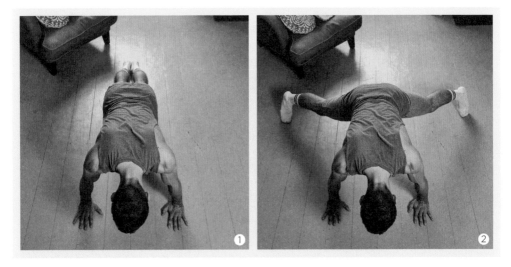

Hamstring curl – slide your feet in towards your bum and back out to starting position.

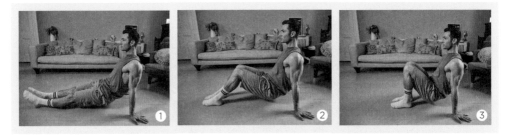

SOCKS ON HANDS

Pec fly – slide your hands out and keep a slight bend at the elbows. I'll be very impressed – or annoyed, because I can't do it! – if you can get back into position 1.

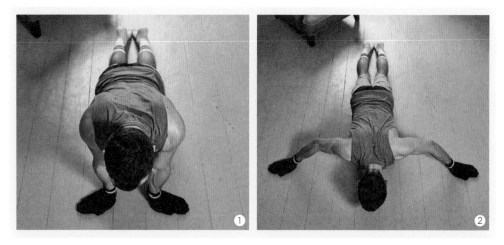

Slide out – keep your knees in the same position and slide your arms out.

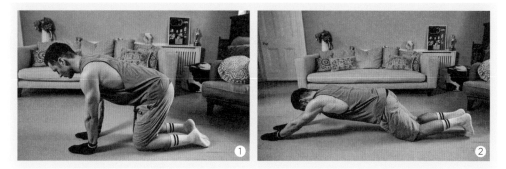

Archer push-up – go into a push-up and slide one arm out to the side. Slide your arm back in on the way up. Alternate. Try this with your knees on the floor to make it easier.

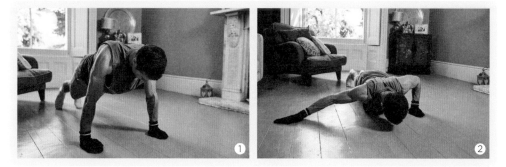

IT'S ALL ABOUT YOU, BABY...

You need to take care of yourself if you have recently had a baby and you should wait until after your postnatal check-up with a doctor at around 6-8 weeks after giving birth before you start taking up any exercise again.

I'm sure any parents though will feel like having young children is something of a workout with all the lifting, bending down and playing that is involved. This isn't so much a workout as a few ways to make the most of always being on the go and getting your body moving whilst also having fun with your little one.

Make sure you perform these exercises with care. Your child will need to have head control and you must always make sure you are in a clear, safe and comfortable area away from obstacles. Listen to your child – this is about making exercise fun for both of you so if they become tired or emotional leave it for another day but even the occasional burst of movement will be good for you both. I'm not sure who's smiling more at the end of this, me or Lola.

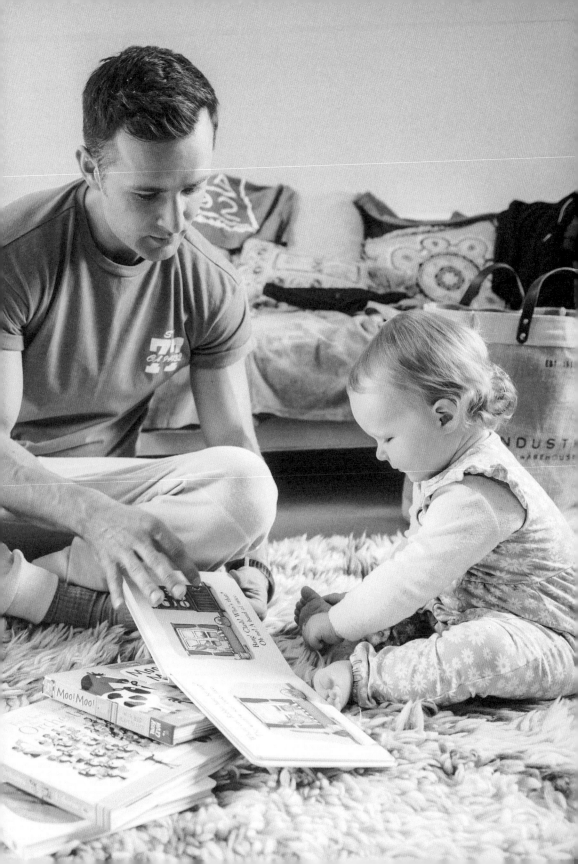

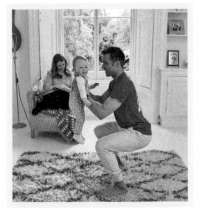

Squat – on a safe, solid floor squat down holding your child close to your body.

Baby twist – if you're just starting out then you can keep your feet on the floor.

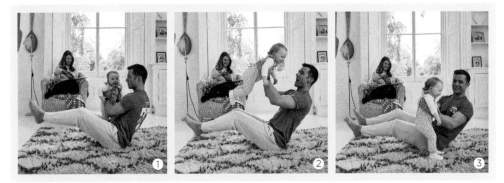

Squat and press – squat down and as you're coming up start to raise your arms.

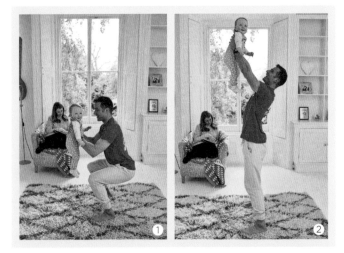

Lunge – add a kiss if they let you!

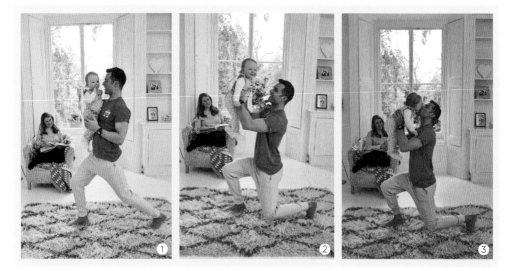

Chest press

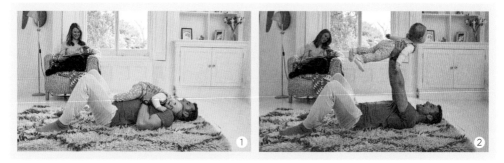

Bear crawl – while chasing your baby. Keep your bum down and your knees just off the floor. Get chasing!

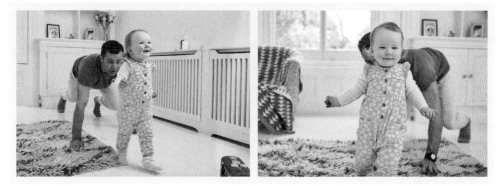

WE ARE
FAMILY

—

Enthusiasm and competitive spirit required! It's interesting to see your level of fitness compared to your kids' – are they going to give you a wake-up call? Either way, exercising as a family is super fun and something we should do more of.

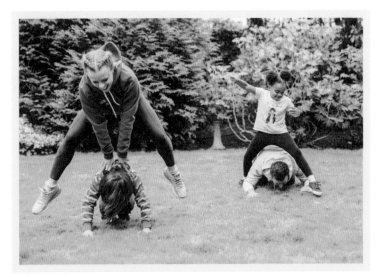

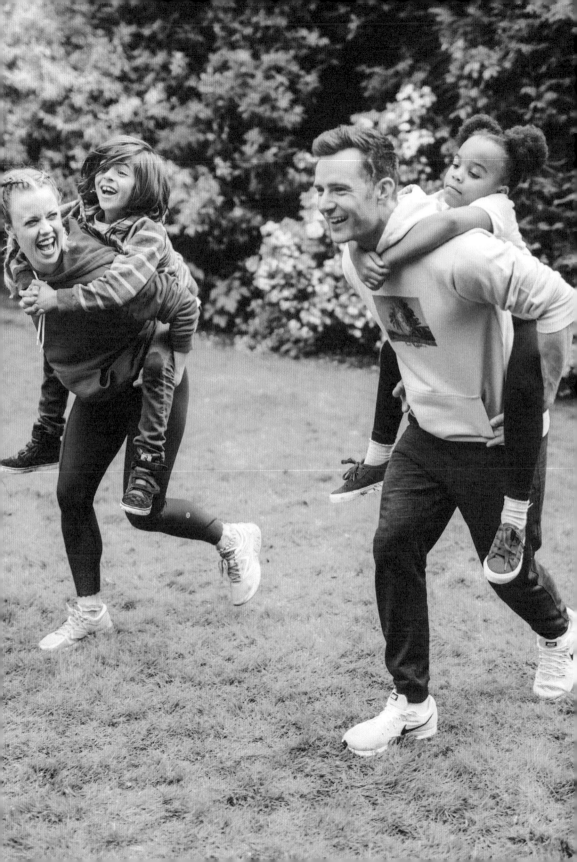

Tag – start with a classic game of tag for 2-3 minutes to get everyone moving and having fun.

Relay races – pair up and let the games begin.

Wheelbarrow across the width of the garden.

Bear crawl back.

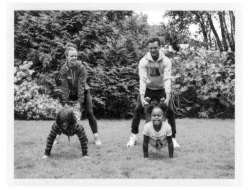 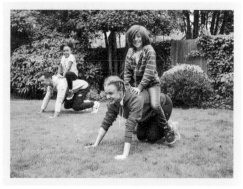

Frog jump across the width of the garden.

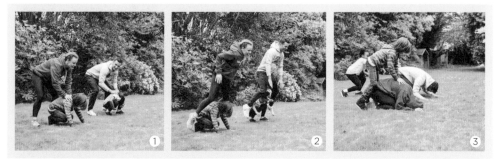

Piggy back back.

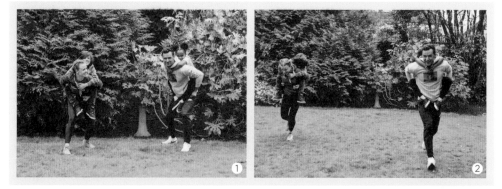

Pike – everyone gets into the pike position. The person on the right end crawls under the others before getting into pike position on the left end. The new person on the right end crawls through and so on until everyone has had their turn.

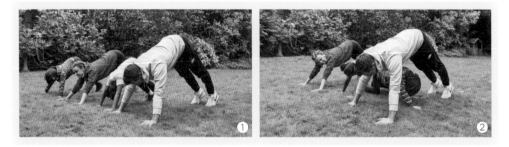

Plank – everyone starts in the plank position taking it in turns to jump over each other.

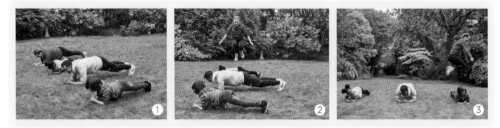

Bear hold – everyone hold with straight arms and bent knees held off the floor whilst one person slaloms around the others. Everyone has a turn.

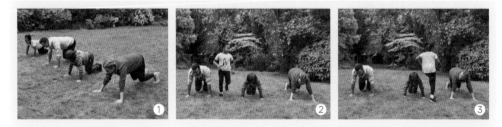

Dish – everyone keeps their heads and feet off the floor whilst one person runs around the group. Everyone has a turn.

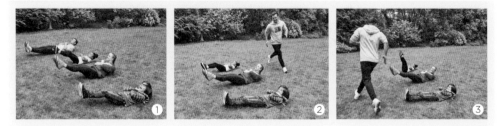

PUSH-UP VARIATIONS

People think of push-ups as a single thing, but there are lots of different types. Push-ups are awesome, because they give you a full-body workout. Here are a few advanced variations for you to try.

Surfer – go down and then push up with an explosive movement and land in a surfing position.

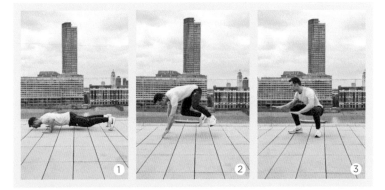

Single arm – before attempting this, work your way up by trying a single arm push-up against the wall or using a table first.

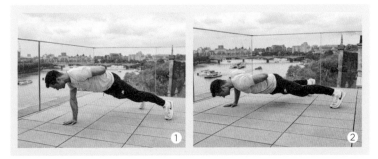

Explosive push-up – start in a wide position and explode on the way up and then land with your hands in a close position. Repeat from close to wide and so on.

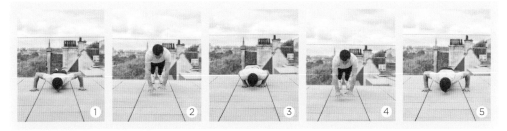

Around the world – create a circular motion as you go up and down.

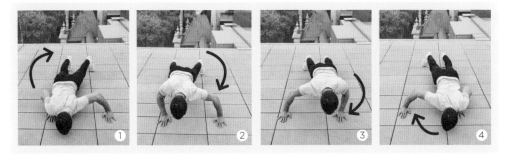

Tricep – keep your elbows tucked in!

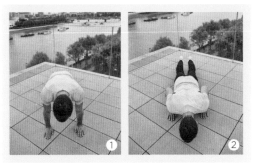

Pause reps – hold your position for a few seconds when you are at the bottom of the push-up.

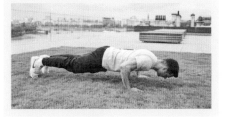

Single leg-up – try ten push-ups with one leg up and then ten with the other leg up for example.

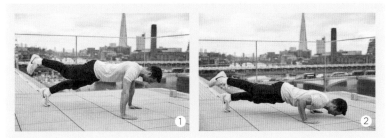

HARD CORE

Aesthetics are, for me, a by-product of exercise. But I still find them an important motivator. This one does what it says on the tin. A strong core is important for all kinds of physical activities and sports. And, don't forget, the core isn't just your abs – it's your back, your obliques, your pelvic floor... I could go on, but I don't want to send you to sleep.

There are lots of different core exercises here and I like to perform what are known as Trisets. Pick three of these core exercises and perform them one after another. Try three rounds of between 10-40 reps of each exercise depending on your ability.

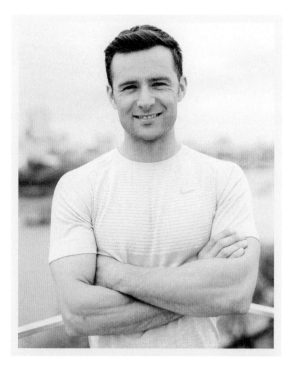

Crunch

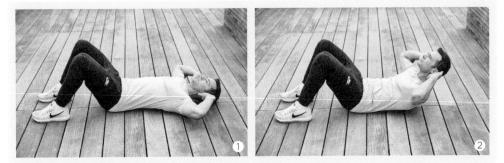

Knees bent crunch

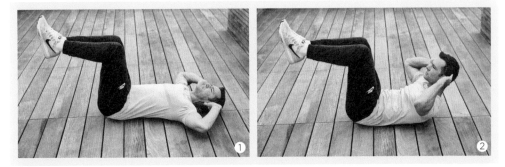

Bicycle crunch – touch your right elbow to your left leg and swap.

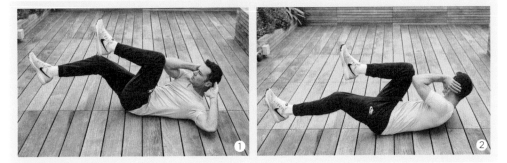

Straight leg raise

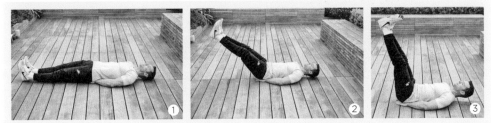

Reverse crunch

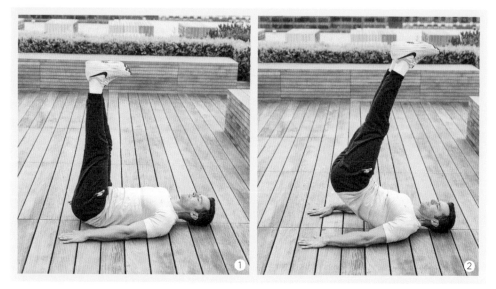

V-sit

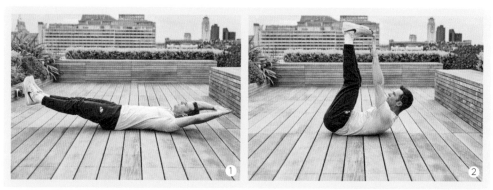

Alternating side leg raise in plank position

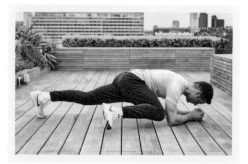

Push-up position leg rotation –
bring your knee to your opposite elbow. Alternate.

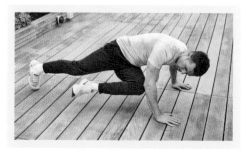

Dorsal raise

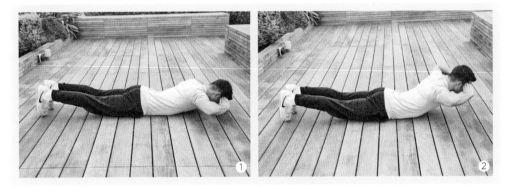

These four are positions that you hold for a length of time.

Side plank – 30 seconds each side.

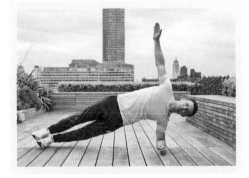

Plank – 30-60 seconds.

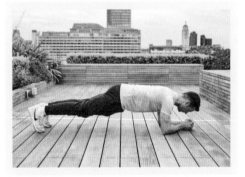

Plank straight arm – 30-60 seconds.

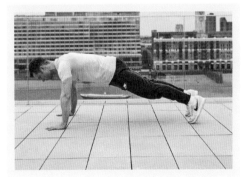

Bear hold – 30-60 seconds.

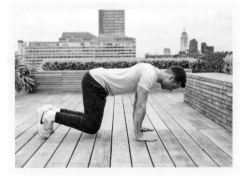

AMRAPS
AS MANY ROUNDS AS POSSIBLE!

———

These are a great way of measuring your progress. The aim of an AMRAP is to repeat the exercises as many times as you can within the allotted time given. The boost to your mood if you manage to get more rounds in than your last attempt is awesome. By now you should be pretty familiar with the most common exercises that make up these workouts. And once you've got to grips with a few of the other exercises in this book, I'd encourage you to come up with your own AMRAPs. Bring your A game – it's you against yourself.

AMRAP LADDER
10 minutes

5 push ups
10 high knees
15 squats
20 mountain climbers

666
6 Minutes

6 burpees
6 push ups
6 alternating jump
  lunges on each leg

CINDY
(a Crossfit AMRAP)
20 minutes

5 pull ups
10 push ups
15 squats

LUCKY 13

———

I came up with this workout when I was on the wattbike doing some intervals. I loved the fact that I'd done exactly 13 minutes (lucky for some). I've adapted it to some bodyweight exercises to make a challenging workout that can be done anywhere by anyone!

'Try moving the exercises around to different time slots to mix it up. To make your intervals more challenging try replacing the rest periods with jogging on the spot.

Squat or squat jump	60 secs
Rest	60 secs
Plank	50 secs
Rest	50 secs
Burpee or chest to floor burpee	40 secs
Rest	40 secs
Knees on floor push-up or push-up	30 secs
Rest	30 secs
Mountain climbers	20 secs
Rest	20 secs
High knees	10 secs
Rest	10 secs
High knees	10 secs
Rest	10 secs
Mountain climbers	20 secs
Rest	20 secs
Knees on floor push-up or push-up	30 secs
Rest	30 secs
Burpee or chest to floor burpee	40 secs
Rest	40 secs
Plank	50 secs
Rest	50 secs
Squat or squat jump	60 secs

STRETCHES

It's very important to cool down and stretch after a workout. There are hundreds of stretches that you can do but here are some of my favourite post-workout stretches. I like to hold each stretch for 20-30 seconds and then repeat.

Calf stretch

Hamstring stretch

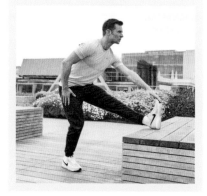

Quad

Hip flexor

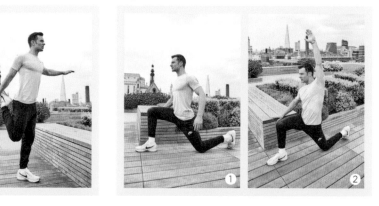

Glute (1st option)

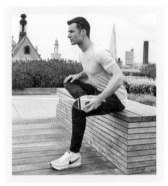

Glute (2nd option)

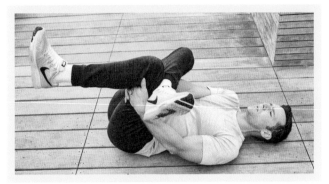

Cobra

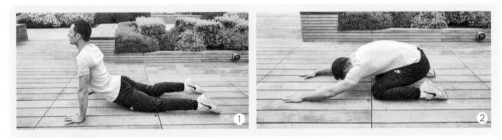

Cross shoulder

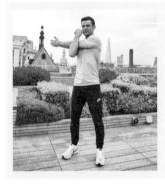

Tricep

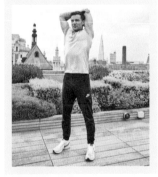

Chest

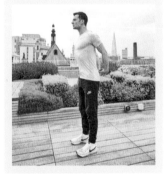

Lats

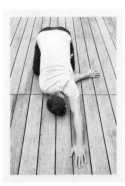

Lower back

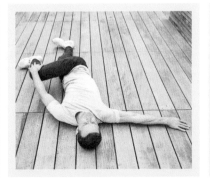

Upper back

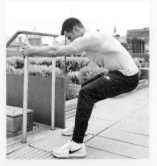

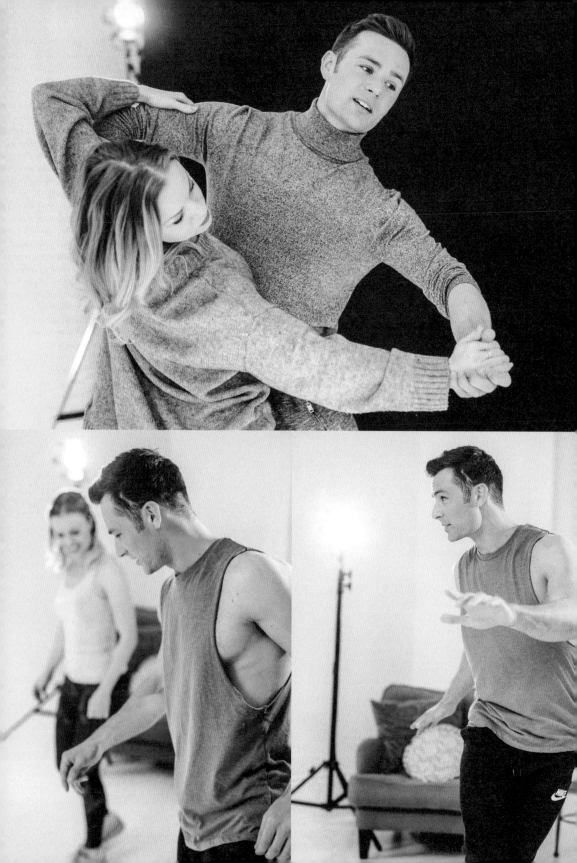

THE
DANCES

—

I had the best time on Strictly and it certainly gave me many great workouts. Dancing is a great way to get moving and a good way to involve all the family. My aim here is to introduce you to some basic ballroom steps as well as showing you a few high energy dances. Some of them (*Do the Twist*, *Jive*, *Can't Stop the Feeling*, *Do You Love Me?* and *Get Happy*) are quite fast and technical so head to youtube.com/HarryJudd for a full run through and some more tips! Keeeep dancing...

WALTZ

When I was on *Strictly*, ballroom dancing was my favourite. My granny particularly enjoyed watching the waltz, so I thought I'd give you some simple ballroom techniques to get you started.
　No matter what your age, it is good to stay active and this might tempt your granny or grandad, or indeed anyone else for that matter, to join you in a bit of exercise.

Ballroom hold – these pictures illustrate what a good hold position looks like.

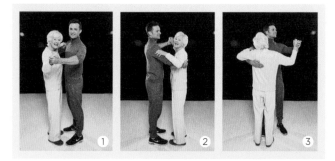

Side to side – in hold position, shift your weight from one foot to the other and sway gracefully from side to side.

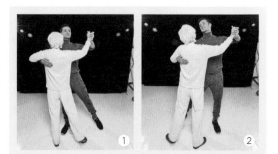

Underarm turn – this is a classic move that we all know. Try starting in hold position and seamlessly move into this underarm turn and back into hold – the beginnings of a dance are starting to take shape.

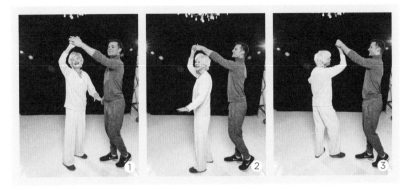

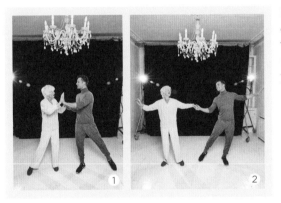

In and out – holding hands with one hand, palms together with the other, separate and step out, rotating your body and extending your arm. Return to starting position.

Forward tap, backward tap – starting in hold position move your left foot forward whilst your partner moves their right foot back. With your opposite foot, tap the ball of your foot gently on the ground keeping your heel raised. Then alternate by stepping back with your right foot and tapping with the left.

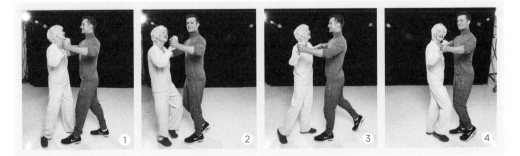

DO THE TWIST

This is a classic, simple dance that anyone can do – and it'll leave you well equipped for the next time you want to bust out some moves at a wedding. My mum particularly likes this one because it works well with songs she grew up with.

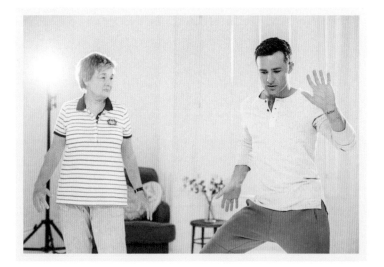

The twist

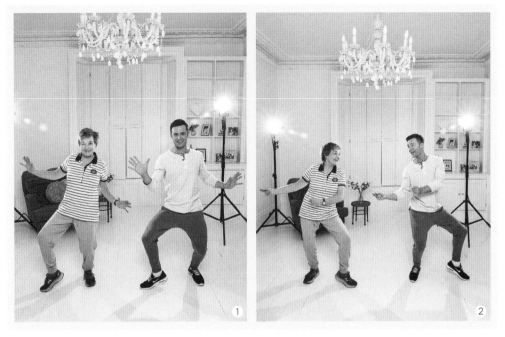

Sit back taps – holding your partner's hand, soften your knees, lean your weight back and tap each foot forward in turn in time with the beat of the music.

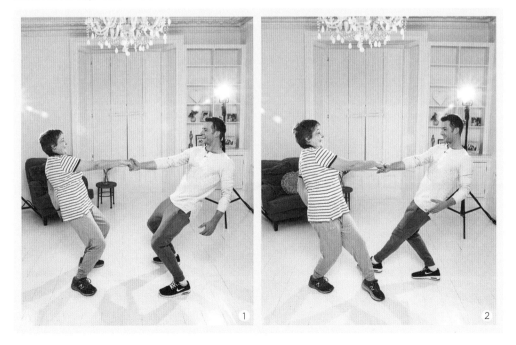

Freestyle – time to drop some of your best moves!

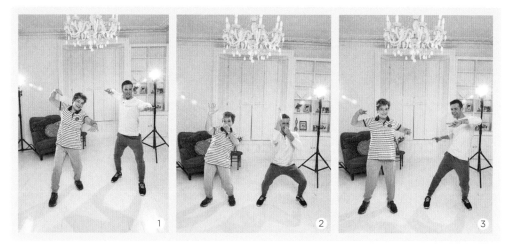

Shake it off – shift the weight onto each foot whilst you shake it off!

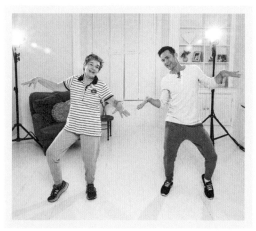

Square claps – clap in the corners of an imaginary square. Land each clap on the beat.

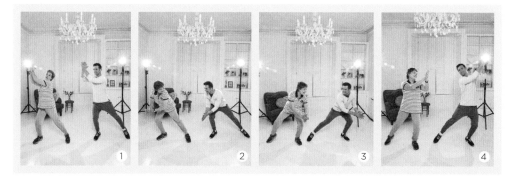

Down and up in build-up – a lot of sixties songs have build-ups (where the dynamic of the song increases). Start low and build up, jump at the top.

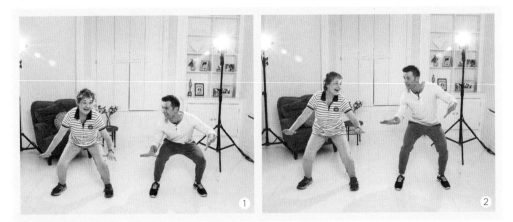

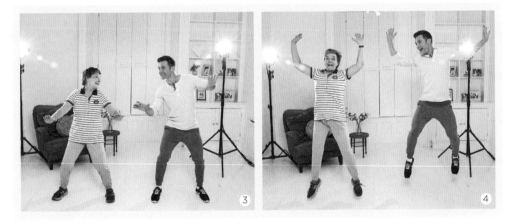

Taps with claps – starting with feet apart, step together and tap one foot and clap. Step apart and repeat on the other foot.

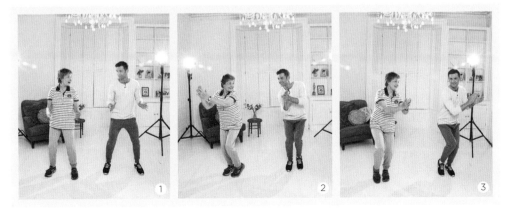

JIVE

—

A jive is a Latin dance and is my favourite Latin dance in ballroom dancing. I did this to 'Greased Lightning' on *Strictly*. (Seeing as I didn't get the part of Danny in Grease at school, I finally got my chance to show off my moves...) This dance is full of fun and energy – and I put it together with 'Runaway Baby' in mind. Enjoy!

—

VERSE 1

Click to the beat

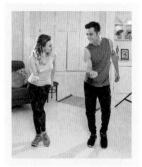

Foot taps to the beat   **Foot taps with arms raised**

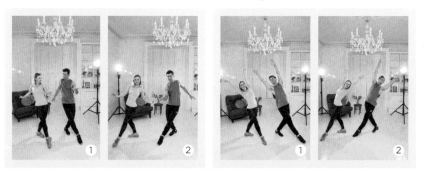

Twist

Leaning twists – as you're doing the twist start to lean your body to the left and then to the right.

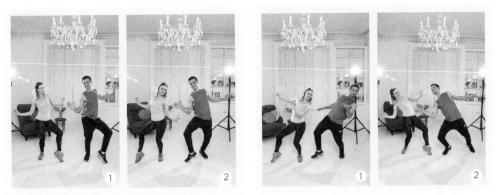

CHORUS 1

Jive kicks – 8 left leg kicks (L), 8 right leg kicks (R), 4L, 4R, 2L, 2R, 1L, 1R.

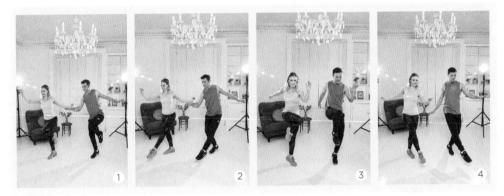

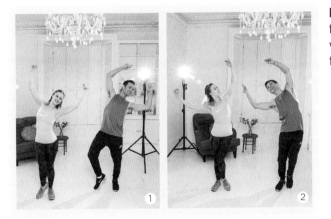

Ponies – skip to the side from one foot to the other whilst leaning towards the foot you land on.

Running on the spot

Stop

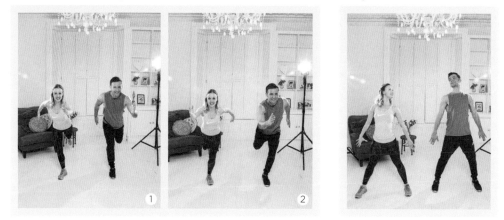

VERSE 2

Clicks

Air piano – or drums!

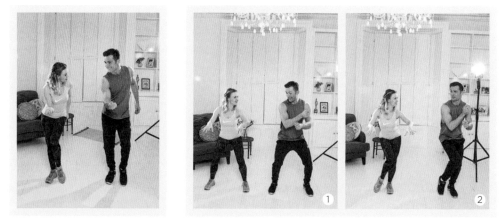

Travelling piano or drums – travel to the side by crossing your feet behind and finish with a foot point and tap. Then travel back the other way.

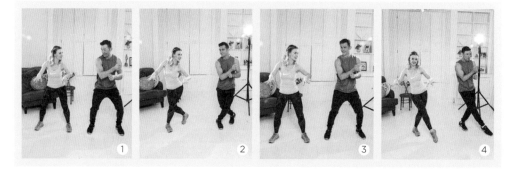

Twist

Leaning twists – as you're doing the twist start to lean your body to the left and then to the right.

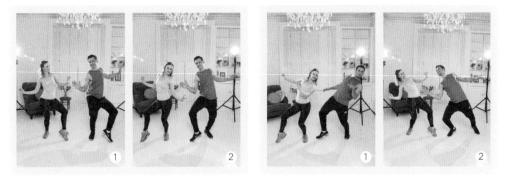

CHORUS 2
Jive kicks – try different combinations of left and right kicks.

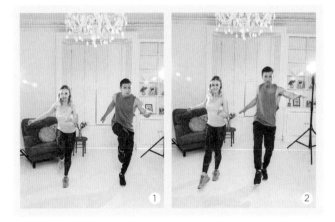

FORWARD 8
Ponies

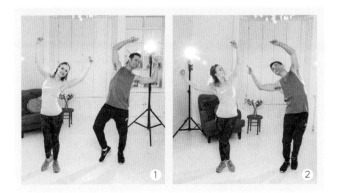

Shoulder roll with a groove – up and down and round and round!

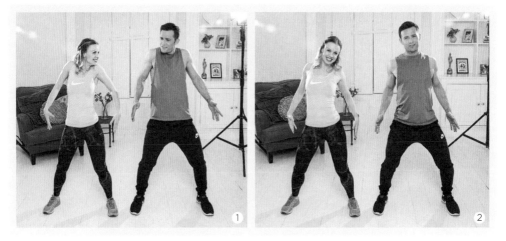

Swinging arms – around with a groove.

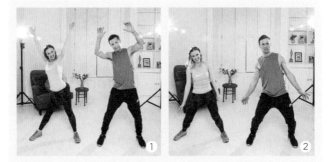

Groove – right then left.

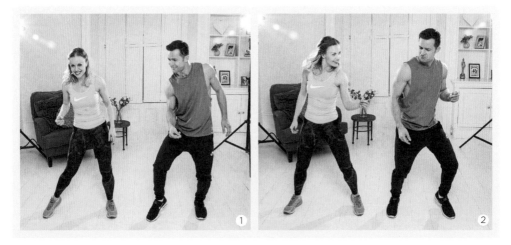

Run

Doubletime run

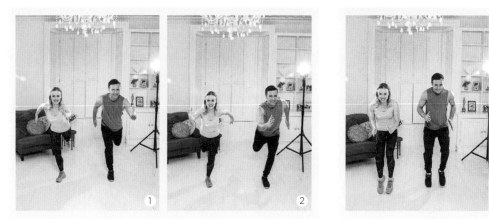

CHORUS 3
Kicks

Ponies

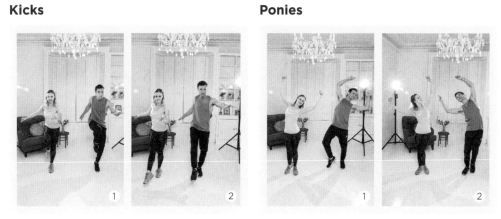

Run

Stop

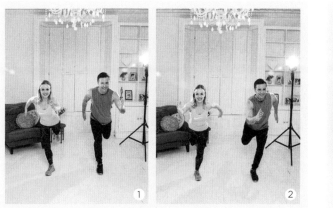
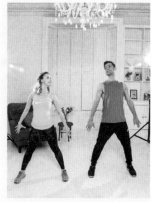

CAN'T STOP THE FEELING

—

I came up with the choreography for this dance to 'Can't Stop the Feeling' by Justin Timberlake and so it is a pop dance with elements of Latin. Don't pretend you don't dance in front of the mirror at home (or is it only me?). Next time you do, you'll have some moves to impress yourself with.

—

INTRO

Clicks and claps – wide and high to the beat. Click when your arms are wide and then clap on the beat.

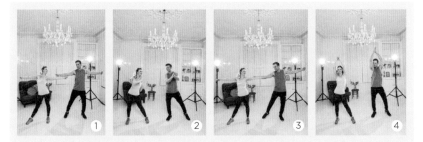

Slide

Stop and drop

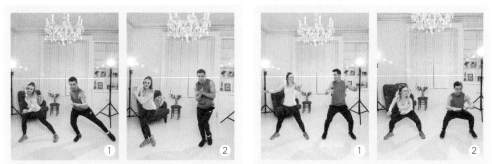

Ronde – to the left and then to the right.

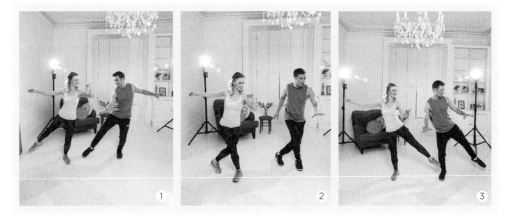

Stop – slowly pulse down with the beat then pulse up and jump into the chorus!

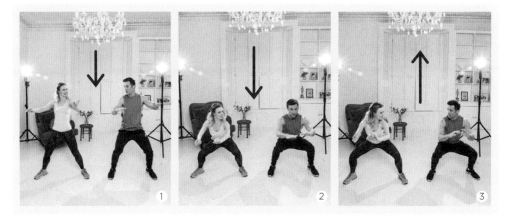

Jumping on the spot

Crazy jumping on the spot

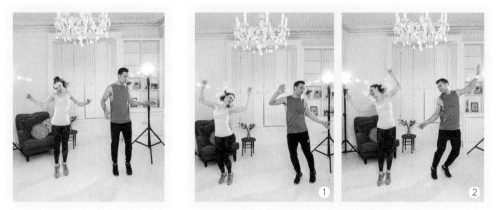

Jumping with a twist

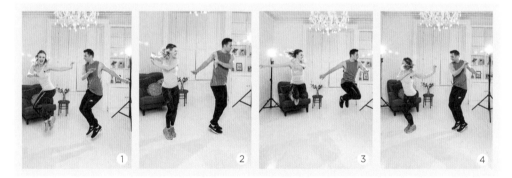

Cross overs

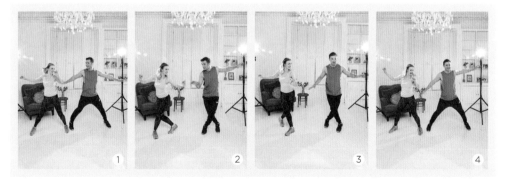

Half-time walk   **Walk on the beat**

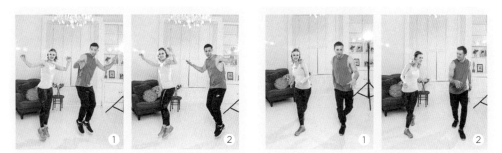

Triple side hops on each side   **Walk on the beat**

VERSE 2
Repeat Verse 1

CHORUS 2
Same as chorus 1 but the end of this chorus is doubled up so after the final walk on the beat I've added in a slide to the right, a slide to the left, a walk on the beat, triple side hops on each side and one last walk on the beat.

MIDDLE 8
Thrusts

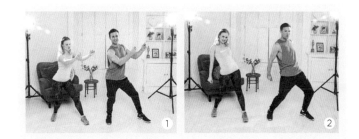

CHORUS 3
Repeat Chorus 2.

OUTRO
Wide and high clicks and claps to the beat – when it's done take a bow!

DO YOU LOVE ME?

—

This is a slightly easier version of the 'Jive' and 'Can't Stop the Feeling' – but just as fun. I like to dance it to 'Do You Love Me?' by The Contours.

—

Side together with clicks – on 'Do you love me?'

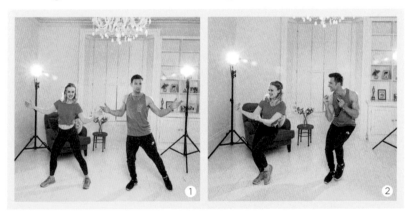

Swinging arms clicks – on 'Now that I can dance'

Stop

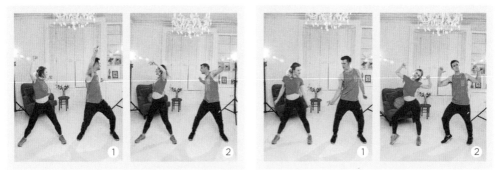

Knees to hands – on each 'work, work'

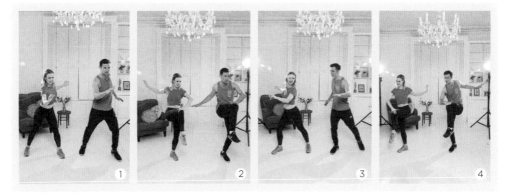

Double claps

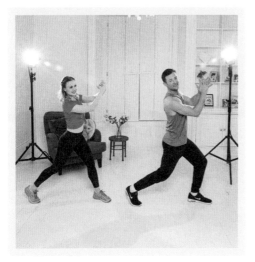

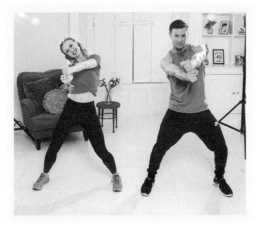

Mash potato – peel and boil the potatoes, add a splash of milk and some butter and get mashing!

Twist

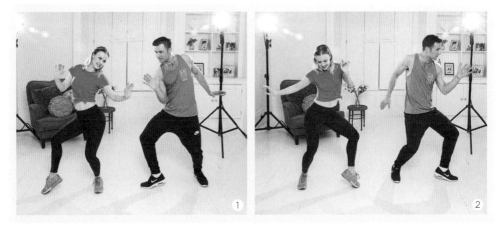

'Tell me baby'

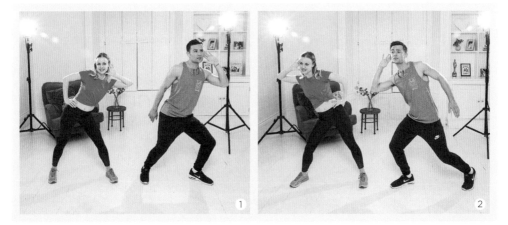

Hip thrust – on 'Do you like it like this'. Well do ya?!

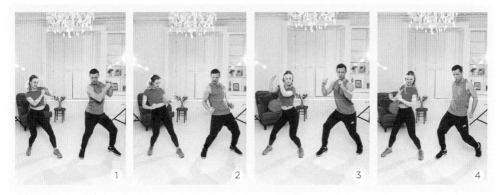

'Tell me baby' – whilst squatting down and up. This is one of those dynamic builds I was talking about

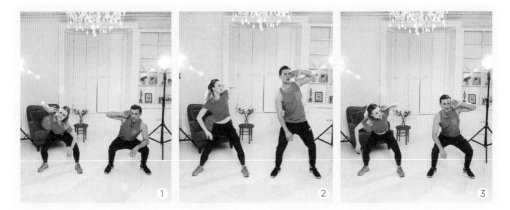

Stop

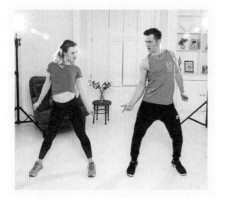

REPEAT

GET HAPPY

—

This is a quickstep style routine choreographed to the song 'Get Happy' that is going to challenge the fittest of you out there. The quickstep was the dance I was dreading the most on *Strictly*, but it's the one people always tell me they really enjoyed. Let me know how your calves feel after this!

—

Ballroom hold

Hop on spot

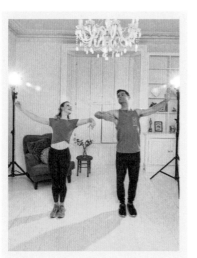 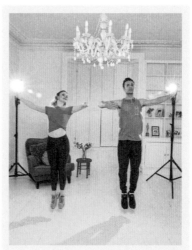

Bell hops
8 each leg, 4 each leg, 2 each leg, 1 each leg.

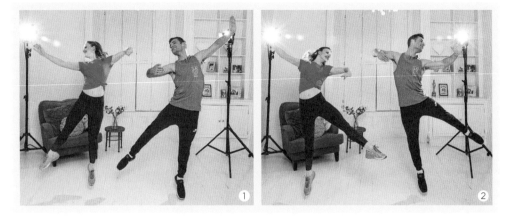

In and outs on an angle – single then double.

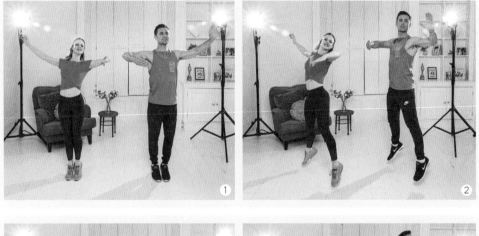

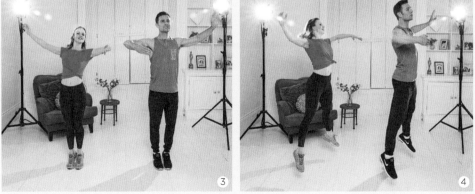

Charleston flicks

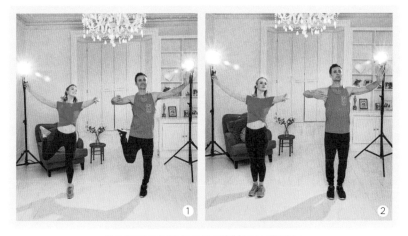

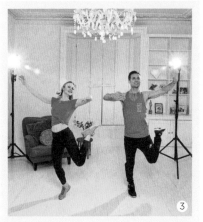

Right kick, feet out, left kick, feet out

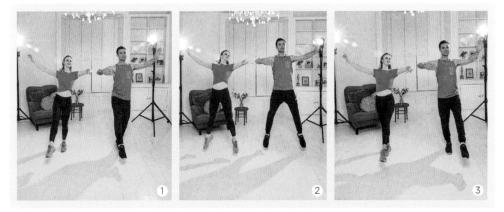

Hop hop slide – both ways.

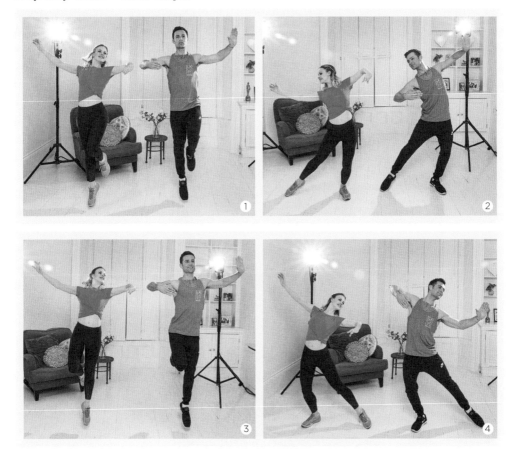

Kick out and slide – kick out with your leg and then bend the same leg in and slide, transferring weight onto the opposite foot. Repeat the other way.

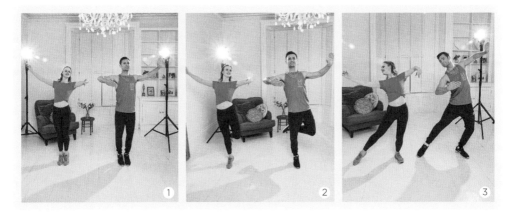

DADDY'S LITTLE PRINCESS

Or Mummy's prince, of course, but this is what I look forward to doing with Lola one day. The grown-up gets to do a workout while the child gets to dance to their favourite music. In this case it had to be a bit of 'Let It Go!' from the *Frozen* soundtrack. Be warned: children are likely to shout 'Again!'

PREPARE

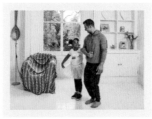

VERSE 1
Slow walk taps – walking forward, tap the opposite foot to the stepping.

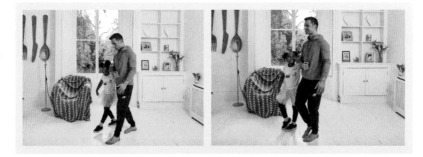

The girl (or person doing the girl's steps) walks around the person in the 'dad' role and jumps over his back leg as he does alternating lunges.

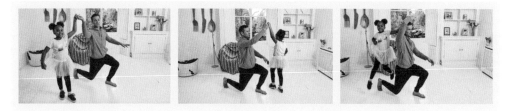

PRE CHORUS
Dad pauses at the bottom of the press-up while the girl jumps over. Dad then pushes up into the Pike position and the girl crawls under.

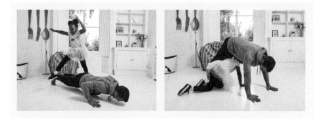

CHORUS 1
Dad lifts the girl up and around, right to left and back again then repeats.

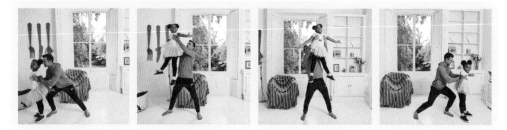

Dad lifts daughter up to the middle and then down low.

Act out cold.

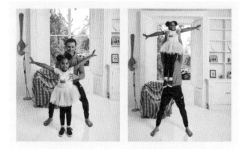

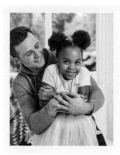

VERSE 2
Skater lunges for dad, while the girl curtseys. Alternate legs.

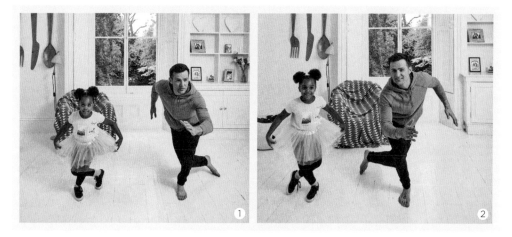

PRE CHORUS
Sit-ups with high fives.

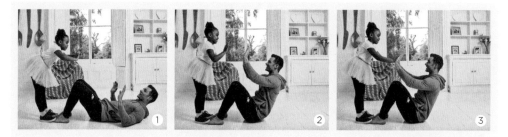

CHORUS 2
Repeat chorus 1.

MIDDLE 8
With dad moving in circles on the floor, the girl runs around in a circle jumping over his legs.

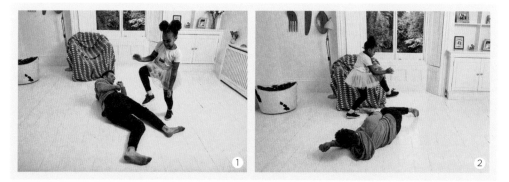

Both dad and daughter do snow angels while dad keeps his head and feet off the floor.

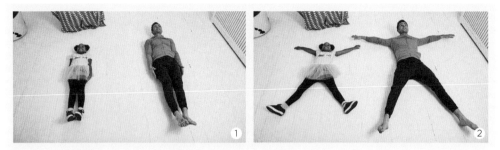

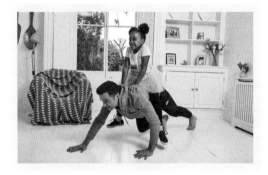

With his daughter on his back, dad bear crawls across the room.

CHORUS 3
Run around (express yourself!), jumping on 'Let it go!'.

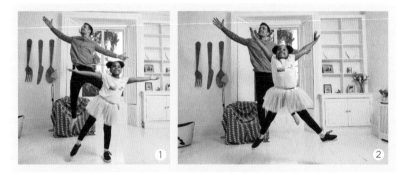

Girl runs into dad's arms for 'Here I am' for 2x squat and press while spinning.

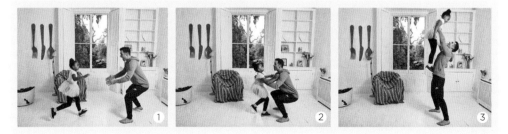

A WORD ABOUT NUTRITION

It will be clear to you by now how much of a difference exercise has made to my life and it is far from just making a difference to how I look. It's about how I feel. It has made me feel happier, it's helped me with my anxiety and my OCD, it has helped me to quit smoking too amongst other things. It has also made a difference to how I eat too.

If you want advice on exactly the right level of protein versus carbs to accompany your workout, I'm afraid I'm not the guy. If you want information on the latest fad diet, look elsewhere. And while it's true that nutrition plays a big part in staying healthy, and that it can be an important complement to exercise, I don't want to overwhelm you. There's plenty of great literature out there about nutrition, and to be honest I just want to try and help to take the stress out of being healthy. If you've done some exercise and are feeling good, I don't want the mood boost to be lost as you stress out about what you should or shouldn't be eating. I'm confident those mood-boosting endorphins will help you make the right decisions anyway.

I take the view that diets mostly have a negative effect, much like unrealistic exercise plans. Okay, so you've lost weight. What happens now the diet is over? Is it sustainable? Probably not. Is trying to stick to it going to make you happy? Probably not. Never mind that extreme levels of weight loss are not good for you. Our goal here is happiness, and I don't think that swinging dramatically between weight loss and weight gain will make us feel remotely positive about ourselves. In fact, the moment I start stressing out about what I eat, I find it brings on my OCD, and I know that's not good for me.

However, of course it is important for our health and general well-being to eat well. So I want to urge you to take a simple, common-sense approach to what you eat. I don't want you to overcomplicate it or stress about it. That way, it can go hand in hand with your physical activity to achieve what you're striving for: feeling great. Here's how I go about it: some simple rules I live by.

I try to cut down on refined sugars and overly processed food, steering clear of fatty fried food and other fast foods. I prefer to think in terms of what I *should* eat, rather than what I *shouldn't*. I eat plenty of fruit and veg – five portions a day is what they tell us, more than that certainly won't hurt, and I always try to have greens with lunch and dinner. Whilst I try not to eat too much red meat, I eat more fish and chicken. I'm something of a carboholic but when I eat things like bread, rice and pasta I always try to go for the wholegrain or wholemeal versions. I drink water like it's going out of fashion.

I don't count my calories or weigh out my macro nutrients. And I constantly remind myself to eat until I am satisfied, not until I am full. I don't let it stress me out. No matter what some people want to make you believe, it really isn't rocket science.

Now, if eating this way sounds like a long way from where you are at the moment, I totally understand. Even when we know what we should or shouldn't eat, it can be tough sticking to it. I have a sweet tooth and I sometimes find it difficult not to succumb!

However, exercise has really helped me in this respect. I have found that it has been the catalyst to me making much better nutritional choices. Before I started exercising, I was way less conscious about what I was eating. When I became active again I started to be more mindful about what I ate and the change in my eating habits was considerable. The Marmite, Philadelphia and cucumber sandwiches accompanied by salt and vinegar crisps and a Dr Pepper that I used to wolf down in the catering rooms backstage on tour went out the window. Now my tour diet is a lot more brown-rice-heavy! Of course we're talking about me here – you don't have to be quite so extreme!

When I've done a bit of physical activity, I find myself wanting to complement it by eating some healthy food. The more healthy food I eat, the more I start noticing the benefits and the better I feel. The more I manage to sustain a better diet, the less I feel like eating unhealthily. I have a very sweet tooth, but trust me the longer you go without sugar, the more unpalatable a bowl of Frosties becomes!

Conversely, if for some reason I can't exercise, I find that my diet takes a hit. I'm more likely to fall back on the foods that I know don't make me feel great. If I have too much sugar, I experience the attendant energy highs and lows, which do nothing for my mood.

Eating properly does take some discipline, there's no doubt about it. However, keeping happy is all about balance. I think it's just as important to treat yourself now and again as it is to eat healthily. That's what I do, a couple of times a week, and it's what I urge you to do as well – although I should warn you that I often wake up the next day feeling a bit groggy and raring to get back to my routine (I call it my sugar hangover!)

Take what you will from these tips but do do this for me: try some of the exercises first and then see what you feel like when it comes to your food choices. If you're anything like me you'll be more inclined to choose the healthier option when your next mealtime comes around.

ACKNOWLEDGEMENTS

To Charlotte Hardman and the Dream Team. You have made the whole process so enjoyable. You have shared my passion and vision from day one and it has kept me focused and determined to get my message out to as many people as possible. You are all not only super hard working but you are all so creative and talented at what you do and have genuinely made this whole experience easier and so enjoyable. I hope to continue working with you in the future. THANK YOU!!!

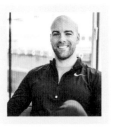

To Adam Jones. As I say in the book, it's always more fun to train with a mate! It's also more fun to work with a mate too. Your training methods are fresh, fun and always challenging. I've loved working and training with you and look forward to beating you in more of our fitness challenges that we pursue in the future! Adam is a personal trainer, sport and exercise physiologist, health and well-being consultant and ante and postnatal exercise coach (adam.parkerjones@hotmail.co.uk and Instagram: @adamjonespt #noshampoojustconditioning)

To Fletch, for constantly pushing me to be better and never allowing me to accept anything but my best. For helping to steer me in the right direction and for always fighting my corner. I genuinely couldn't have done it without you.

To Nikki, for all your hard work and patience. Especially when I call and email you without realising it's the weekend! You keep all the plates spinning and make it look easy.

To the Clifton girls, Karen and Joanne, for lending me their gift for dancing during the making of this book. Your work ethic is inspiring and your energy and love for dance is infectious. You've made me look better at dancing than I am so thank you!

To Dr Dance, for sharing your story. A truly inspiring tale of adversity conquered through a love of dance. Thanks for you enthusiasm — it's catching and I hope to spread your dance love in this book.

To Dr Zoe Williams, for sharing your experiences with me. Not only are you inspiring young girls with your story, you've inspired me. Awesome to meet a real-life gladiator!

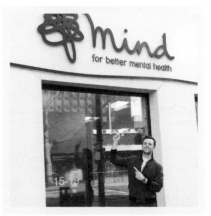

To Mind, for meeting with me. The work you do saves lives and gives people a shot at happiness. Thank you for being so happy to help me with my mission! For anyone looking some advice or more suggestions on different ways to help please do check out www.mind.org.uk

To Professor Sharma, for sharing your expertise with me. I hope my book does justice to the passion that you have for helping people through exercise.

To The Lean Machines (@theleanmachines), Roger Frampton (@rogerframpton), Hannah Tyldesley and Emily Kier (@twicethehealth), Tameka Small (@tamekasmall), Zanna Van Dijk (@zannavandijk), Carl Richey (@teamrichey), Jasmine Cabourn (@wanderlust_pochahontas), Jamie-Ray Hartshorne (@jayrayfitness), Rachel Evans (@healthyandpsyched), Jon Weston-Stanley (@healthyjon), Courtney Pruce (@courtneypruce), Ban Hass (@banhass), Charlotte Thomas (@lungesandlycra), Jemma Thomas (@mummas_health_hub), Doug Armstrong (@epiphanized) and James Stirling (@london_fitness_guy) for all their support and encouragement.

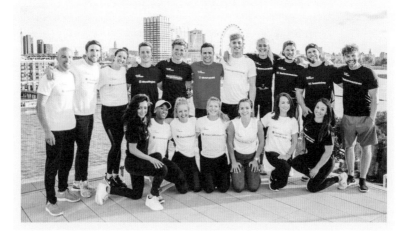

To Dave Spearing, for keeping it real and not pre-ordering the book.

To Adam Parfitt, for helping me put my thoughts into words. We always laugh when we write and that's a huge reason why this whole process has been enjoyable. Thank you for sharing my passion on this subject and for helping me to shape this book.

To Mum, for your continuing and unfaltering support. You always say yes when I ask for your help and you always bring a smile! Your warmth and enthusiasm never go unnoticed.

To all the other people who have helped me in so many ways: Will Speed*, Fiona Rose*, Alice Morley*, Heather Keane*, Emma Knight*, Rosie Stephen*, Ruth Ferrier, Nathan Burton, Dan Jones, Sophie Fox, all the accommodating Hodder folk who took time out of their day to get sweaty with me in an office aerobics session, Derek Bremner (www.derekbremner.com), Bob Bennett-Baggs, Summer Brooks and Tobias Ungelson and the team at Sylvia Young, Tessa Landers, Nadine O'Toole, Anna Thompson, Rosalind Keep, and everyone at St Ninians School. (*Dream Team!)

And finally to Izzy, for supporting me through this whole process. It's been a long project and you've always given me the space and time to achieve what I set out to achieve. You, Lola and bump are my everything and I do it all for you.

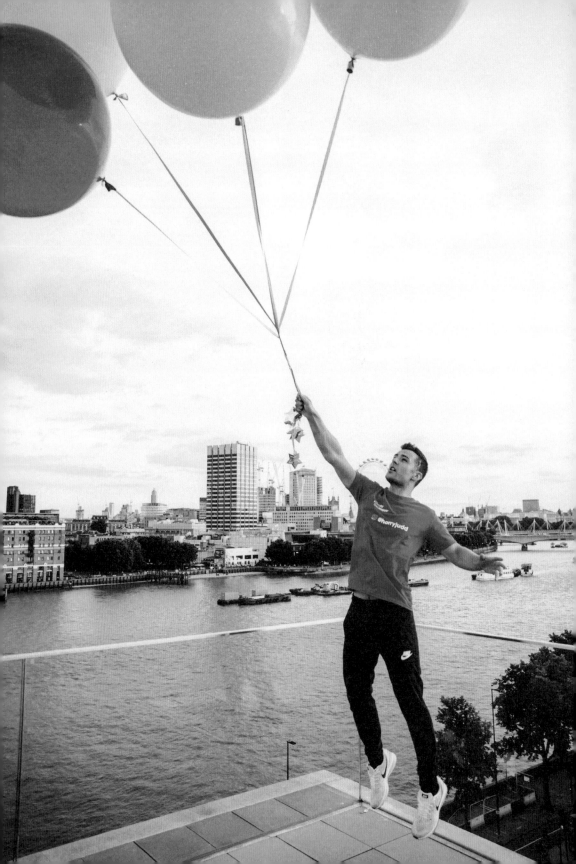

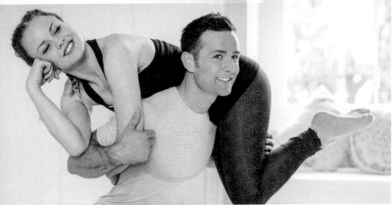
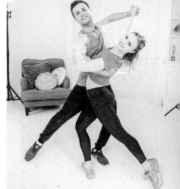
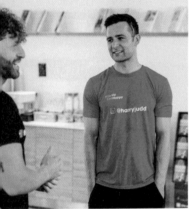
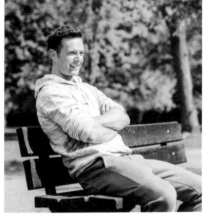
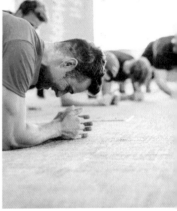
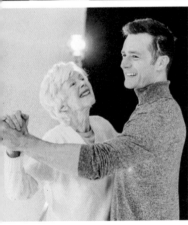
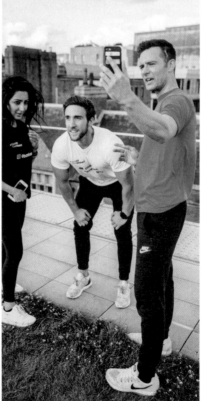
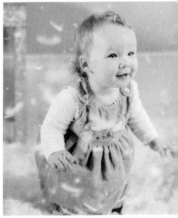
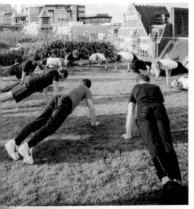
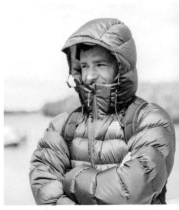